OCCUPATIONAL THERAPY IN RHEUMATOLOGY

CRPYK

FORTHCOMING TITLES

Occupational Therapy for the Brain-Injured Adult
Jo Clark-Wilson and Gordon Muir Giles

Physiotherapy in Respiratory and Intensive Care
Alexandra Hough

Understanding Dysphasia
Lesley Jordan and Rita Twiston Davies

Management in Occupational Therapy
Zielfa B. Maslin

Dysarthria
Theory and therapy
Sandra J. Robertson

Speech and Language Problems in Children
Dilys A. Treharne

THERAPY IN PRACTICE SERIES

Edited by Jo Campling

This series of books is aimed at 'therapists' concerned with rehabilitation in a very broad sense. The intended audience particularly includes occupational therapists, physiotherapists and speech therapists, but many titles will also be of interest to nurses, psychologists, medical staff, social workers, teachers or volunteer workers. Some volumes are interdisciplinary, others are aimed at one particular profession. All titles will be comprehensive but concise, and practical but with due reference to relevant theory and evidence. They are not research monographs but focus on professional practice, and will be of value to both students and qualified personnel.

Occupational Therapy in Rheumatology

An holistic approach

LYNNE SANDLES
Principal Occupational Therapist
The Dene Centre
Newcastle-upon-Tyne Council for the Disabled

CHAPMAN AND HALL

LONDON • NEW YORK • TOKYO • MELBOURNE • MADRAS

UK	Chapman and Hall, 2–6 Boundary Road, London SE1 8HN
USA	Chapman and Hall, 29 West 35th Street, New York NY10001
JAPAN	Chapman and Hall Japan, Thomson Publishing Japan, Hirakawacho Nemoto Building, 7F, 1-7-11 Hirakawa-cho, Chiyoda-ku, Tokyo 102
AUSTRALIA	Chapman and Hall Australia, Thomas Nelson Australia, 480 La Trobe Street, PO Box 4725, Melbourne 3000
INDIA	Chapman and Hall India, R. Seshadri, 32 Second Main Road, CIT East, Madras 600 035

First edition 1990

© 1990 Lynne Sandles

Typeset in 10/12pt Times by Mayhew Typesetting, Bristol
Printed in Great Britain by St Edmundsbury Press Ltd,
Bury St Edmunds, Suffolk

ISBN 0 412 31560 2

British Library Cataloguing in Publication Data

Sandles, Lynne
  Occupational therapy in rheumatology: an holistic approach.
  1. Man. Joints. Arthritis & rheumatic diseases. Therapy
  I. Title   II. Series
  616.7206

  ISBN 0 412 31560 2

Library of Congress Cataloging-in-Publication Data

Sandles, Lynne.
    Occupational therapy in rheumatology : an holistic approach /
  Lynne Sandles. − 1st ed.
      p.   cm. − (Therapy in practice series : 19)
    Includes bibliographical references.
    Includes index.
    ISBN 0–412–31560–2
    1. Rheumatism–Patients–Rehabilitation. 2. Occupational
  therapy. 3. Holistic medicine. I. Title. II. Series.
    [DNLM: 1. Occupational Therapy. 2. Rheumatic Diseases–
  rehabilitation. WE 544 S217o]
  RC927.S26   1990
  616.7′2306515–dc20
  DNLM/DLC
  for Library of Congress   90–2589
                                                                  CIP

Contents

Acknowledgements

The completion of this book has been achieved with the support, advice and contributions of many people. I would like to express my thanks to all those who have been involved in any way. Special thanks go to Jo Campling and Chapman and Hall and to Helen Jones for her endless patience and help.

This book would not, however, have been written without the people of the North East of England who have shared freely their experiences, their humour and made me welcome in their homes. They are the people from whom I have learnt rheumatology and I dedicate this book to them.

Preface

This book is written primarily for occupational therapists and occupational therapy students but will be of relevance to anyone working with clients with rheumatoid disease. It is hoped that the text will communicate the challenge faced by therapists to establish management programmes appropriate to the identified needs and priorities of the individuals with whom they work, the potential to utilize a wide range of skills and the opportunity to contribute to the understanding of the many unanswered questions which remain in relation to rheumatic diseases.

The aim of this book is to present an holistic approach to the management of rheumatoid disease, considering first, the ways in which rheumatoid disease can affect a person's life and then looking at the approaches and techniques used by therapists to minimize these effects. This approach has been chosen as it is fundamental to both the philosophical basis of occupational therapy and the management of a chronic progressive disease. An holistic approach considers the physical, psychological, social and spiritual aspects of a person and the ways in which these have been effected by an underlying disease process. Each of the components are interrelated, illustrating the complexity of establishing appropriate management programmes and evaluating their effectiveness. The first two chapters consider the effects of rheumatoid disease on clients and their families.

An holistic approach identifies the need for a diversity of skills to be available to both the therapist and client. The range of approaches and skills needed in rheumatology often extends the boundary of the conventional multi-disciplinary team and crosses from a hospital setting into the community and from a ward environment into the laboratory. To function as an active team member therapists must have an understanding of the work of other members. Thus rheumatology offers therapists the opportunity to extend the base of their knowledge and the potential to work within a team offering a diversity of skills. Chapter 3 considers the holistic approach to management and the multi-disciplinary team.

Assessment is a fundamental component of establishing management programmes enabling areas of need to be identified and prioritized goals to be set and providing a baseline from which the effectiveness of interventions can be measured. Many of the techniques used by therapists in the field of rheumatology remain unevaluated. The need to gain insight into the effectiveness of interventions is great and opportunity to contribute to the knowledge base of rheumatology is there for anyone who wishes to take up the challenge. Evaluative procedures apply not only to establishing the needs of clients but also to the work of therapists. The process of assessment is considered in Chapter 4.

The chronic progressive nature of rheumatoid disease poses enormous challenges to clients in relation to learning new skills to adapt to their changing circumstances. The amount of time that therapists spend with clients is fractional in terms of the overall duration of the disease. This coupled with the increasing demand from clients to be active participants in their management programmes leads therapists to work with a variety of educational approaches on both an individual and group basis. Chapter 5 considers different approaches to conveying information, increasing client involvement and assisting clients to cope with change.

The final section of the book considers specific interventions used by occupational therapists in hospital and community settings.

It is hoped that this book will convey the wide horizons open to therapists working within rheumatology and identify many of the, as yet, unanswered questions. This field of medicine offers both breadth and depth. The challenge of rheumatology is working with individuals and individual responses to a chronic progressive disease. There is no such phenomenon as a treatment programme for rheumatoid disease and it is this factor which extends the skills of therapists to their maximum in relation to both clinical work and research.

1

Introduction to the chronic arthritides

STRUCTURE OF DIARTHRODIAL JOINTS

Joints which possess a synovial-lined cavity are called diarthrodial joints. They comprise a variety of types of cells and structures. The articular surfaces of bones are covered by cartilage and lined by synovium which is normally approximately three cells thick. Some synovial cells secrete synovial fluid into the joint cavity, others are phagocytic. The subsynovium is formed from a matrix of collagen, proteoglycans and elastin; these molecules, secreted by fibroblasts, provide synovium with its strength and flexibility. The tissue contains also blood vessels, adipose cells, nerves and lymphatics. Cells from the circulation pass through synovium, thus a few leucocytes can be seen in the connective tissue of normal joints. Tendons or ligaments may insert into bones near joint margins at a site called the enthesis.

TYPES OF CHRONIC ARTHRITIS

The chronic arthritides involve tissue destruction and persistent inflammation in one or several joints. Little is known about what environmental factors are important for inducing tissue damage in joints. Presumably most people are exposed to most of these factors, but relatively few develop arthritis. The nature of the individual's response, by inflammation and immune cell activation, to tissue damage is probably of central importance in determining which people are able to heal and repair tissue and which develop further tissue destruction and hence disease.

Most types of chronic polyarthritis are multisystem diseases. In other words, the brunt of damage and inflammation is borne by joints but other tissues are involved remarkably often. Indeed,

1

Figure 1.1 Diagram of a diarthrodial joint

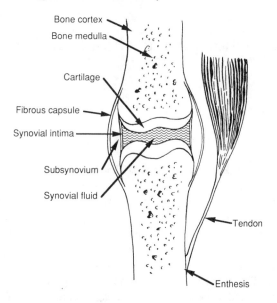

clinical manifestations of the involvement of other systems may precede or follow the onset of joint disease by many years and it is important to recognize that the symptoms and signs of these diseases may evolve with time. Sometimes the disability that arises from involvement of other systems is more debilitating for the client than that of the arthritis itself, and is occasionally life-threatening.

The main clinical basis for distinguishing one type of arthritis from another lies in the distribution of joint involvement. However, although characteristic patterns of joint involvement are described for different types of arthritis it is often the case that individual clients do not exhibit such classical patterns. In these circumstances an open mind must be kept regarding diagnosis and careful repeated examination may reveal a diagnosis at a later date when other features of the disease have developed. The initial clinical assessment of a client involves making a diagnosis, based upon the distribution of joint involvement and of systemic features, determining the extent to which the disease interferes with his or her life and gauging the nature of the client's response to the problem. Usually this assessment can be accomplished with the minimum of laboratory investigation.

The salient features of the four most common types of chronic polyarthritis are described below.

Figure 1.2 Distribution of joint involvement in osteoarthritis

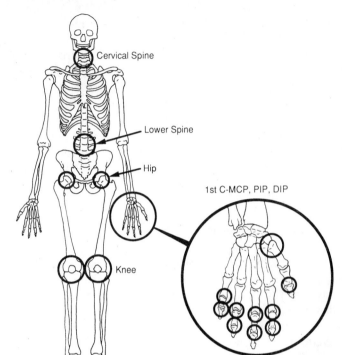

Osteoarthritis

Osteoarthritis is the most common of the chronic arthritides. It occurs as either a mono- or polyarthritis and can involve the spine, hips and knees and is characterized by cartilage degeneration and osteophyte formation. Peripheral joints can also be involved, in particular, the distal and proximal interphalangeal joints, the first carpo-metacarpophalangeal joint and the first metatarsophalangeal joint.

The clients often have bony swellings of the distal interphalangeal joints, called Heberden's nodes, and of the proximal interphalangeal joints, called Bouchard's nodes. Although osteoarthritis may have no accompanying systemic manifestations, it develops frequently in patients with certain rare conditions such as acromegaly and ochronosis.

3

The predominant symptoms are pain and loss of function. Pain may originate from the joints themselves or, when disc prolapse from the vertebral column occurs, from nerve roots at sites of exit from the spinal cord. Loss of function may be attributed to the pain of inflammation or, in the later stages, to joint destruction and deformity. However, a remarkable degree of function is often retained in knee or hip joints which appear by their radiological appearances to be affected severely. Clients may obtain benefit from measures aimed at improving general levels of fitness, such as losing weight, but once symptoms have developed they rarely resolve completely. However, if progressive joint destruction does occur it usually does so only slowly. If disability becomes severe, hip or knee joint replacement may be indicated.

The crystal related arthropathies

A variety of types of crystal have been found in inflamed and damaged joints. Monosodium urate crystals have been known for many years to be associated with gout, a disease which manifests either as repeated acute attacks of monoarthritis (classically involving the first metatarsophalangeal joint) or as a chronic destructive polyarthritis often accompanied by renal impairment.

The factors which promote the deposition of urate crystals in tissues are understood poorly although concentrations of uric acid in the serum, which are high in some clients, probably contribute to this. Several diseases, such as haematological malignancies, and several drugs, such as diuretics, are known to increase serum uric acid concentrations and precipitate gout. Uric acid is the end product of a biochemical pathway by which endogenous and dietary purines are metabolized. The drug allopurinol inhibits an enzyme which is active in this pathway, namely xanthine oxidase, and thus prevents the production of uric acid. Allopurinol is used to treat clients who suffer frequent attacks of acute gout or who have associated renal impairment.

Calcium pyrophosphate crystals can also be found in joints in association with acute attacks of arthritis, usually in the knees. Clients may be perfectly fit between attacks. Interestingly, crystals can be deposited in asymptomatic joints because it is quite common to observe radiologically calcification of the joint cartilage, an appearance termed chondrocalcinosis. This shows that the deposition of crystals in joints does not necessarily result in arthritis, but at

Figure 1.3 Distribution of joint involvement in rheumatoid arthritis

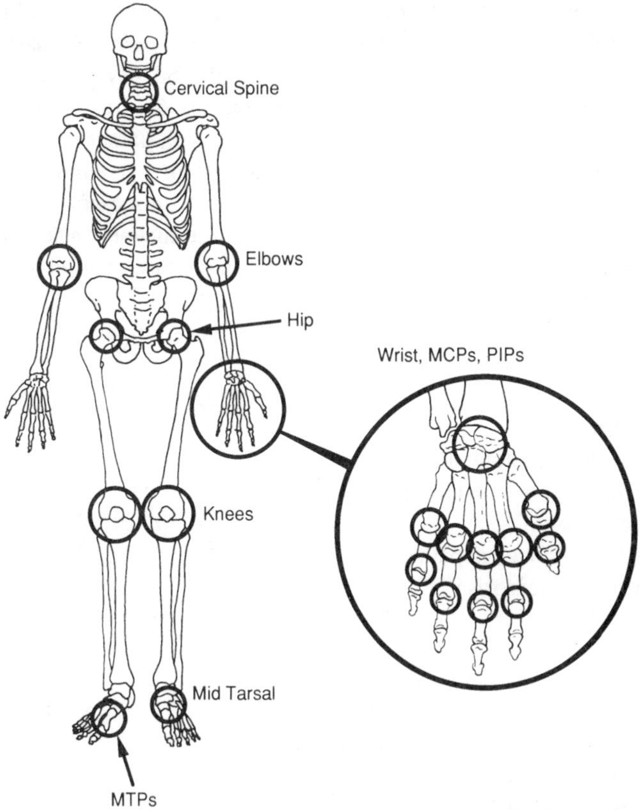

present the other mechanisms which determine the pathogenicity of crystals are not understood. It is rare for rapid or severe joint destruction to be associated with crystal deposition alone and if it occurs the presence of other types of arthritis should be considered. Management is based upon explanation and encouragement to improve general levels of fitness and function. Simple analgesics or antirheumatic drugs may be beneficial during acute attacks.

Rheumatoid arthritis, Sjogren's syndrome and related diseases

Rheumatoid arthritis is characterized by a chronic, destructive, peripheral, symmetrical polyarthritis, often associated with subcutaneous and tendon nodules.

It can develop at any age, including childhood. There is marked systemic involvement, with malaise, weight loss, anaemia and lymphadenopathy, and involvement of other systems resulting in vasculitis, neuropathies, pulmonary and ocular disease. In particular, clients frequently suffer from a dry mouth and dry eyes, and this complex of clinical features is known as Sjogren's syndrome. Sjogren's syndrome is also associated with other multisystem diseases (such as systemic lupus erythematosus, systemic sclerosis, polyarteritis nodosa) and organ-specific diseases (such as Hashimoto's thyroiditis, Graves disease, pernicious anaemia) and many clients develop these other conditions before or after the onset of rheumatoid arthritis.

The following is a list of common extra-articular features of rheumatoid arthritis.

1. Systemic
   (a) Rheumatoid nodules
   (b) Sjogren's syndrome
   (c) Anaemia
   (d) Lymphadenopathy
   (e) Amyloidosis
   (f) Vasculitis;
2. Ocular
   (a) Scleritis and episcleritis;
3. Neurological
   (a) Peripheral nerve entrapment
   (b) Cervical cord compression
   (c) Peripheral neuropathy;
4. Pulmonary
   (a) Pleurisy
   (b) Pleural effusion
   (c) Pulmonary fibrosis;
5. Cardiovascular
   (a) Pericarditis and myocarditis
   (b) Pericardial effusion.

One prominent feature of these diseases is the chronic activation of immune cells some of whose responses are directed towards different proteins in the body. Hence, these diseases are known collectively as autoimmune diseases. Many clients with rheumatoid arthritis have high concentrations of antibodies called rheumatoid factors in their serum. Rheumatoid factors, which are found in many diseases of chronic inflammation and whose pathogenic significance is unclear, bind antibodies of the IgG subclass. The term seropositive is used to denote those clients with raised titres of rheumatoid factor in their serum.

In addition to the distribution of joint involvement, two other features of rheumatoid arthritis are striking. First, for reasons which are unknown the disease is more common in females. Second, it is frequently the case that over several generations more members of a family develop rheumatoid arthritis or a related condition than would be expected by chance, suggesting that genetic factors contribute to disease pathogenesis. One region of the genome known to be important in pathogenesis is known as the HLA region. The proteins encoded by genes in this region play a role in the induction of immune responses. One of the genes in the HLA region is called the DR gene, and in some groups of clients with rheumatoid arthritis there is a higher prevalence of individuals with DR4 or DR1 haplotypes than in the population as a whole. It is unresolved at present whether DR genes themselves play a role in pathogenesis, or whether other genes close to them are in some way responsible.

The principal symptoms of rheumatoid arthritis are joint pain and swelling, with stiffness in the mornings or after prolonged immobility. The severity of rheumatoid arthritis characteristically undergoes periods of exacerbation and remission, the pattern of which is unpredictable and probably unique for each individual client. Broadly speaking, in some clients complete resolution occurs after months or years, others experience a persistent disease of fluctuating severity whilst relatively few suffer relentlessly progressive disease. At any stage, any of the associated clinical features may supervene and be associated with deterioration in the client's condition. Changes in the client's symptoms may also reflect the fact that their ability to cope varies according to changing personal circumstances. The extremely variable natural history of rheumatoid arthritis is reflected in the spectrum of histological and radiological changes seen in the joints. The characteristic histological features are of synovial hypertrophy and hyperplasia with infiltration of tissue by inflammatory and immune cells. The joint cavity is filled with an inflammatory exudate. Where the synovial tissue spreads over cartilage it is called 'pannus'. Changes occur in the adjacent bone and cartilage leading to erosion of these tissues and hence destruction of the integrity of the joint. Chronic inflammation and tissue damage in associated structures, such as tendons, contribute to the characteristic clinical features and to the patient's disability.

Any client with rheumatoid arthritis has a unique and complex combination of physical, social and psychological disability, each component of which varies to different degrees at different times. In order to set management goals which are optimal and attainable it is essential that each person contributing to the care of the client appreciates all aspects of his or her condition.

The aim of management is to maintain the maximum possible level of function. The approaches adopted in order to attain this vary from client to client and a skillful management team will ensure that all potentially useful resources are deployed appropriately. Much time needs to be spent, particularly in the early stages, in discussion and explanation with the client, the family and often with other individuals important in their lives. It is vital that the client be given correct advice about methods for maintaining joint function, since most can expect the severity of inflammation to diminish at some stage but loss of the range of movement in a joint may prove irreversible. Medical treatment for co-existent extraarticular disease may be necessary, but the use of anti-rheumatic drugs is given much less prominence in modern medical management. Concerns about side effects, lack of efficacy and increased joint destruction in the long term have probably all contributed to this changing view. A similar changing view pertains regarding the use of intraarticular steroid injections. For clients with severe destructive joint disease, joint replacement may be indicated and this should be performed, if possible, before marked deterioration in function occurs. Throughout, the management team and the client should be aware of the general importance of maintaining his or her morale in order to meet the challenge of this chronic disease.

Ankylosing spondylitis and related diseases

Ankylosing spondylitis characteristically involves the sacro-iliac joints and the spine and probably develops as a result of chronic inflammation primarily at entheses.

Although the severe systemic upset which is such a marked feature of rheumatoid arthritis is not found in ankylosing spondylitis, it is nevertheless common to find involvement of other systems in these clients. Again, these features can develop at any stage of a client's disease.

Common extra-articular features of ankylosing spondylitis are listed below.

Figure 1.4 Distribution of joint involvement in ankylosing spondylitis

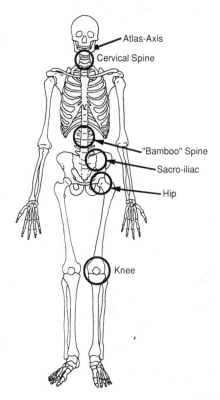

1. Ocular
   (a) Uveitis and conjunctivitis;
2. Pulmonary
   (a) Upper lobe fibrosis;
3. Cardiovascular
   (a) Aortic regurgitation
   (b) Conduction defects;
4. Neurological
   (a) Nerve root or cord compression;
5. Systemic
   (a) Amyloidosis.

Certain other diseases (notably psoriasis, psoriatic arthritis, inflammatory bowel disease and Reiter's syndrome) occur in clients with ankylosing spondylitis and in their families more often than would be expected by chance. The HLA region makes an important genetic contribution to the pathogenesis of ankylosing spondylitis because in caucasian populations over 95% of clients have the HLA B27 haplotype compared to about 8% of the population as a whole. It is important to remember, however, that the HLA B27 haplotype is not a high risk factor for disease and most people with this haplotype are healthy. Despite much research the mechanism of HLA B27-disease associations is still unclear. It may be that the HLA B27 gene itself, or its encoded product, or a gene in close proximity, mediate this effect.

The symptoms of ankylosing spondylitis develop in adolescence or early adult life. Although it was thought previously to be more common in males, clearly it has been underdiagnosed in females and probably occurs equally in both sexes. The principal symptoms are of low back pain and stiffness, the presence of stiffness helping to distinguish it from other causes of low back pain such as nerve root inflammation or vertebral collapse. Quite often there is arthritis in one or more peripheral joints also. In ankylosing spondylitis, as in rheumatoid arthritis, there is an infiltration of inflammatory cells at sites of disease together with chronic activation of immune cells. As in rheumatoid arthritis, some of the immune response is directed towards the body's own proteins such that ankylosing spondylitis is also regarded as an autoimmune disease. In contrast to rheumatoid arthritis, however, the chronic inflammation in ankylosing spondylitis leads to fibrosis and then marked calcification, a process which can result in severe and characteristic spinal deformity with loss of spinal mobility.

It is now well-recognized that the single most important aspect of management is for the client to undertake a regular programme of exercises in order to prevent the disastrous loss of spinal mobility which occurred in clients in the past. The potentially catastrophic consequences of spinal immobility should be emphasized repeatedly. Although some clients undertake such exercise programmes themselves, following initial instruction, many take the opportunity to perform them in groups and this probably contributes usefully in other ways to support and maintain morale. Some clients find antirheumatic drugs useful at times when the disease is active but the continual and habitual ingestion of drugs should be discouraged. For clients with severe joint destruction, hip or knee joint replacement can be performed.

LABORATORY AND RADIOLOGICAL ASSESSMENTS

The most important aspect of diagnosis is the clinical history and examination. There are very few circumstances in which investigations are of central importance for diagnosis, although they are used in clinical practice for monitoring disease progress or determining the extent of multisystem involvement. In interpreting results of investigations for these purposes, the rate of change over time for the various parameters is often as important as their absolute values. Some commonly-used investigations are discussed below.

Parameters measured in peripheral blood

The erythrocyte sedimentation rate (ESR) is the simplest and most widely used objective measure of severity of inflammation. The ESR increases in the presence of inflammation anywhere in the body and therefore is not a specific indicator of arthritis. The ESR depends to a large extent upon the concentrations in blood of a variety of different proteins (such as C-reactive protein, $\alpha 2$ macroglobulin) which are secreted from cells such as hepatocytes during inflammation but whose functions are unclear. In clients with rheumatoid arthritis blood platelet concentrations increase with disease severity.

Haemoglobin concentrations characteristically fall in clients with chronic disease, although other possible causes of anaemia (such as blood loss or haemolysis) must be borne in mind. Decreases in blood haemoglobin, platelet or white cell counts may also indicate drug toxicity.

Biochemical investigations provide information on the function of different organs (for example, urea and electrolyte concentrations reflect kidney function) and indicate generally the state of activation of the immune system, as measured, for example, by serum concentrations of immunoglobulins, complement components and cytokines. Many clients with rheumatoid arthritis have high concentrations of rheumatoid factors, which are antibodies which themselves bind to antibodies of IgG type. Again, none of these measurements have absolute diagnostic specificity for any particular type of arthritis.

Parameters measured in synovial fluid

In arthritis, synovial fluid contains a variety of types of inflammatory cells and biochemical mediators of inflammation. At present, however, the only two circumstances for which examination of the fluid is of accepted diagnostic value are (i) to look for crystals in suspected crystal deposition diseases; and (ii) to culture for bacteria if infection is suspected.

Radiological investigation

X-rays are used for diagnosis, to monitor disease progress, and to help determine strategies when joint replacements are planned. X-rays illustrate the degree of joint destruction but often correlate remarkably poorly with function. It is interesting to note that clients with severe inflammation do not necessarily develop severe joint destruction whereas clinically mild inflammation may sometimes be associated with marked damage to bone and cartilage. The radiological changes reflect the pathological processes occurring in the joints. For example, in rheumatoid arthritis the early changes are seen in peripheral joints with narrowing of the joint spaces and periarticular osteoporosis. This may be followed by erosion of bone and cartilage, and subsequently by complete loss of the structure of the joint. In ankylosing spondylitis the first radiological changes (which may take years to develop) are seen as blurring of the margins of the sacroiliac joints. This may be followed by sclerosis and accompanied by characteristic changes in the spine, reflecting the inflammation and calcification which occurs in spinal joints and ligaments.

SUMMARY

Advances in biochemistry, immunology and molecular biology are continually providing exciting new insights into mechanisms of inflammation and immunity. It is hoped that one day these will lead to successful methods of curing, or even preventing, chronic arthritis. For the foreseeable future, however, the management of these conditions will depend upon the ability of carers to address the complex needs and demands of clients and their families. Rheumatology remains therefore one of the most challenging and interesting specialities in clinical medicine.

FURTHER READING

R. Cailliet (1982) *Soft Tissue Pain and Disability*, F.A. Davis Company,

J.S. Pigg, P.W. Driscoll, R. Caniff (1985) *Rheumatology Nursing, A Problem Orientated Approach*, Wiley Medical Publications.

G.K. Riggs, E. Gall (1984) *Rheumatic Diseases, Rehabilitation and Management*, Butterworth Publishers, Guildford.

2

Psychosocial aspects of rheumatoid disease

The unique response of individuals to illness is an indication that aspects, other than the underlying disease process, can influence the way in which a person responds to and experiences symptoms of a disease and the ways in which that disease can affect a person's lifestyle.

Management of a chronic progressive disease can only be effective when the psychological and social implications of the disease are considered alongside the physical symptoms, no one factor can exist in isolation.

> In rheumatoid arthritis, as with other illnesses, a unique interaction exists between disease, stages in life, personality and environment. (Rogers *et al.*, 1982)

The uniqueness of this interaction presents a challenge to any professional working in the field of rheumatology as no standard treatment or regime can be implemented. Clients' responses will be different, they will develop their own coping mechanisms, have varying levels of motivation and place different values on aspects of their lives.

The interaction between these different facets is not only varied from individual to individual but will also vary for each individual during the course of the disease. The variability of rheumatoid disease means that a client is passing from periods of exacerbation to periods of remission and from periods of acute illness to periods of chronic disease. This leads to the responses of clients having to be flexible to cope with varying levels of pain, functional ability, deformity and the psychosocial impacts of these variations. The added problem of feeling controlled by, as opposed to controlling, the disease can also arise. A high degree of unpredictability, change and feelings of loss of control can lead to stress and anxiety.

Healthcare professionals need to gain an understanding of these interactions in order to help clients identify and develop coping strategies which are appropriate to their needs and those of the environment in which they are functioning.

In considering the psychosocial aspects of rheumatoid disease this chapter will consider some of the relationships between the disease process and self-concept, stages in life and the environment and how these factors can be interrelated.

SELF-CONCEPT

Self-concept is a collective name for various aspects of 'self' relating to the way in which we perceive ourself and our relationship to the environments in which we exist. Thus this concept comprises many facets each of which is ascribed a value and an emotive component and is based upon previous experience. The self-concept is not a static concept as components may change, highly valued attributes may become less valued and new components may be incorporated.

The onset of a chronic disease can pose a considerable threat to self-concept and lead to varying degrees of stress and anxiety. Rheumatoid disease can lead to fundamental changes in a client's self-image and role. The ability to cope with these threats will depend upon the client's ability to utilize a range of coping strategies. Decreased self-esteem, depression and a sense of loss of control can result if a client is unable to utilize coping strategies to deal with such threats to their self-concept.

Some of the components of self-concept will be discussed in greater detail and consideration given to the way in which rheumatoid disease can effect them.

Self-image

Self-image refers to the way we perceive our body looks and functions and the emotions that our body generates, therefore it has both a visual and an emotive element. The body schema, or visual map, is developed in early childhood and represents the development of a physical image, this image develops throughout life as our body undergoes change, especially during such periods as adolescence. As this physical picture is developing an emotional component is developing alongside it. The emotional component is influenced

15

largely by societal influences which impose positive and negative values to aspects of appearance. These values start to form at an early age and can be seen in school playgrounds where any child who is overweight or looks different is often the focus of harsh ridicule. Positive and negative images are exploited and reinforced daily by advertising agents who spend vast amounts of money on projecting the desirable image to which we should all aspire, one which is usually portrayed alongside other symbols of glamour, wealth and good fortune. Thus positive and negative messages are received about appearance and the social acceptability of the way we perceive our body to look.

The wish to conform to these perceived socially acceptable norms is strong and the strength of the media, which is brought daily into our homes via papers, magazines and television, creates pressure to aspire to the 'socially acceptable image'. The consequences of not fitting into this image can include withdrawal from social situations, low self-esteem, isolation, stress and anxiety.

If members of the public, or indeed health care professionals are asked to describe the image of a person with rheumatoid disease words such as 'deformed, gnarled hands' and 'twisted joints' are used frequently. If the public image of a disease is one which is associated with deformity this can figure highly on the list of anxieties of a person who has been newly diagnosed as having rheumatoid disease. The familial link of rheumatoid disease may also mean that clients have observed at close quarters the progressive nature of the disease and be all too aware of the possibilities of developing deformity.

Fear of the onset of deformity is expressed frequently by clients and yet it is questionable how much time is spent by professionals on discussing this problem. Perhaps this is because the onset of deformity is seen as an inevitable consequence of the disease process about which little can be done. It is interesting, however, when talking to clients, the profound effect an altered appearance can have on their function, especially the social consequences. On an individual level we can identify how much a positive self-image can increase confidence in social interactions and influence other peoples' perception of us: 'Looking good, feeling great' is a frequently used phrase.

While in reality there may be little that can be done by therapists to prevent the development of deformity, it is necessary to consider the ways in which poor self-image can affect a clients' function and ways in which these effects can be minimized. Isolation and social withdrawal may be a consequence of pain or limited mobility but may equally be the result of embarrassment about appearance or gait. Therapists need to consider ways in which clients can be helped to cope with the threat to their body image and ways in which they can draw attention away from their visual deformities, and develop their self-confidence in social interactions.

Incorporated within self-image is sexual identity which refers to a person's awareness of themselves as a sexual being in relation to other people. A change in self-image can effect sexual identity and the way in which people perceive their ability to form or maintain sexual relationships and to both give and receive sexual satisfaction. The impact of a chronic disease on a person's sexuality will vary from client to client. A young single person may feel that their ability to form a relationship with another person is threatened; 'Will anyone find me attractive?' A mature person in a relationship may worry about their partner's changing attitude, they may believe they are no longer sexually attractive or that an inability to maintain previous levels of sexual function may lead their partner to seek fulfilment else where.

Three components of rheumatoid disease have been identified as affecting a person's body image, these are:

1. the disease process;
2. treatment programmes;
3. perceptions (Smith *et al.*, 1985).

Disease process

The disease process, which progresses often towards deformity, is an area, which in the early stages of the disease is often a cause of conflict for many clients. The onset of deformity is acknowledged as a source of anxiety but the implications of the disease in its early stages, having little apparent visual deformity are often neglected by therapists, this will be discussed under 'perceptions'.

The disease process can affect a person's self-image in several ways. The amount of time and energy devoted to appearance may lessen due to fatigue and lack of energy. Self-care skills may be cut to the minimum in the mornings due to the amount of time taken for morning stiffness to wear off and the extra time needed to complete activities. Limitation in movement and weakness of grip may lead to difficulties in carrying out activities and if people have become dependent in self-care skills the priorities of a carer may not be the same as those held by the client and attention to detail may not be as great. Clients whose mobility has become impaired may be reliant upon members of the family or other carers to buy clothes, make-up etc. on their behalf, losing control, to some extent, over the image which they wish to project. Clients with limited upper limb function may be unable to style hair or apply make-up and feel that the ability of their husbands to assist in these matters is limited. Environmental barriers may make access to hairdressers, dentists, health clubs etc. impossible.

The development of deformities such as swan neck and boutonniers deformities and ulnar drift are difficult to conceal and gait may be affected by lower limb deformities such as fixed flexion and valgus deformities of the knees. The development of deformities can lead to a change in a person's self-image as they can feel their deformities to be very apparent and attracting unwanted attention. This can lead to withdrawal from social situations and alterations in interpersonal relationships.

The degree of distress a person feels about changes in their appearance does not necessarily correlate with the degree of deformity they have developed. What may be perceived by one person to be a mild deformity which causes little stress may be perceived by someone else as unacceptable and be the cause of much stress. A young woman attending a self-management course was extremely distressed by the sight of other peoples' hands within the group. She was a telephonist receptionist and was desperate to do anything which may prevent deformities developing in her hands. Other group members did not all share her concern and were more worried by some of the other implications of the disease. She found the confrontation with other group member's deformity so distressing that she felt unable to attend more than the first session. Her priority was to seek assurance that her hands would not become deformed and she was desperate to do anything possible to prevent deformities occurring.

Non-verbal communication is an important aspect of any interaction providing information, cues and feedback and is fundamental to communication. The impact of deformity on non-verbal communication has not been addressed in relation to rheumatoid disease but is worth considering. Hands are an essential component of the communication process adding graphic detail to language, providing a visual portrayal of emotions such as anger, frustration and anxiety, and via touch expressing affection and providing sensory stimulation. A person who feels their hands to be unsightly and incapable of giving pleasure or their actions to be clumsy may be concealing one of the most receptive and expressive forms of non-verbal communication.

Visual deformity can also determine the type of response a client receives in a social situation, 'seeing the wheelchair before the person'. Clients relate how they have to develop the social skills to cope with the responses of other people to their visual deformity, trying to project their personality over the visual perception and value judgements that have been made as a consequence of it.

Treatment programmes

It should be acknowledged that some of the treatment programmes prescribed will also have an affect on a person's self-image. Medication can cause changes in appearance, both in the short term as a result of adverse reactions and in the long term resulting in such changes as the moonshaped face seen in clients who have been undergoing prolonged use of cortico-steroids. Scarring after joint replacement surgery or the healing of an ulcer can be distressing and cause embarrassment to some clients. One young client had stopped going swimming with her friends following joint replacement surgery because she was embarrassed by the scars she had on her legs. Coming to terms with an altered body image can take a long time and the amount of confidence needed to carry out an activity such as swimming in public baths should not be under estimated. Some clients will overcome this by going to swimming sessions organized specifically for people with disabilities where they hope to find more understanding but this can cause conflict between being categorized as 'disabled' and 'different' or carrying out a valued activity.

The use of assistive equipment, splints and orthopaedic shoes will provide a visual marker of a disability and may draw unwanted attention. The design of many orthoses is a cause of conflict for clients who may have to choose between accommodating such things into their self-image, to obtain pain relief or increased function, or coping with the pain and limitations in order to maintain their self-image. Some clients will opt for the latter which is one of the reasons for items being stowed in cupboards when taken home. It is only when the advantages of using the equipment or orthoses outweighs the effect on the self-image that a client will adapt their image to accommodate the change.

One of the most frequently expressed losses, in relation to appearance is the ability to wear fashionable shoes. 'No matter how much effort I put into my clothes and make-up I always look down and see great clod-hoppers on my feet'. If it is felt that appliances have a therapeutic value that is aimed at the prevention of deformity this issue must be addressed. It is a false expectation to believe that clients will wear unsightly orthoses and appliances, unless it is absolutely essential, and says little for the value given by professionals to the body image of the clients with whom they work.

Perceptions

A person's perception of themselves as handicapped depends on many factors one of which is their self-image. In the early stages of the disease-process a client has very few visual deformities and this will influence the way in which society reacts to that person. A clinician may, on examination, identify synovitis, or careful observation may highlight a protective gait or posture, but these manifestations of pain and stiffness are usually not observed by people such as work colleagues, members of the public and families, therefore conflict can arise for the client.

In *Disability and Disadvantage*, David Locker (1983) describes the process of 'legitimation' which is the process by which society acknowledges a person as having a disability. The public image of arthritis is usually associated with old age and gross deformity, therefore when confronted by a young person with no apparent sign of deformity, legitimation of the disease becomes more difficult. Hidden handicaps are more difficult for society to legitimate. This point is emphasized by the experience of a young mother in the early stages of rheumatoid disease who was going through a period of remission except for one ankle. Her leg had been placed in a below knee walking plaster to rest the joint. During the time that her leg was in plaster she received more offers of assistance than she had ever experienced, despite, apart from the one joint, experiencing less pain and functioning at a greater level of independence than over the last year. A person with a visual clue of handicap is automatically identified as 'disabled' and their limitations and handicaps acknowledged.

Conflict arises for the person with no visual deformity between appearing no different and therefore not being perceived as 'disabled' and thus attracting unwanted attention, sympathy etc., and yet having some limitations and possibly being in need of some assistance and support in certain situations. One young mother abandoned her full shopping trolley in a supermarket when she approached the checkout for disabled people and was told to use another because that till was only for the use of people with a disability. This conflict can be ongoing as clients may strive to maintain what they perceive as an appearance of 'normality' despite being aware of limitations and changes in appearance and sometimes wanting those limitations to be acknowledged.

This conflict was summarized recently by one client as she was adjusting the beautiful scarf she used to conceal her collar; 'I have my pride and my vanity, I want to look good, but the more I try to keep up my appearances the less people believe me when I say I am not feeling too good. "Oh but you look wonderful they all say". At times I could scream.'

The concept of self-image is central in rheumatology highlighting possible areas of conflict, stress and anxiety. It is an issue which may arise throughout the course of the disease as a clients' self-image and their functional abilities change. A poor self-image can lead to a person withdrawing from situations which evoke and reinforce feelings of 'standing out in a crowd' or act as a reminder of 'what I used to look like'. Catching a glimpse of a reflection in a shop window can be very distressing, as small mirrors at home do not give a full reflection of outward appearance, posture and gait. It can also lead to isolation in a social sense and within personal relationships. Conflict between wanting to appear 'normal' and yet gain some acknowledgement of needs can be a cause of anxiety.

A very clear insight into the emotive struggle associated with a changing body image was provided by one client who made several points worth reiterating. The first was that while she knew her outward appearance had changed, especially as she often used a wheelchair, when she dreamt, the image of herself she saw was of a person who was still fully ambulant and physically the same as before the onset of her disease. Dreams like these were distressing as they seemed to provide a constant reminder to her of what she used to look like and throw back in her face any hope that she had started to come to terms with her new appearance. She also related how she forgets the visual image that other people see, so that when friends and family can see from her expression, or pallor that she is exhausted or in pain she still thinks she can bluff them by joking, laughing and playing the fool. 'I forget that people can see what I look like because I avoid looking in a mirror or a window and so

I have never seen what I can look like when I am struggling to stand up or do something. On the inside, to me, I look no different than I ever have done and forget that other people can see the reality rather than my fantasy – I am on the inside looking out.'

The same client provided a graphic description of how she had tried to cope with accepting that her legs were no longer going to function in the way in which they used to. She had been very sporting and active and was trying to come to terms with having to use a wheelchair for long distances, an altered gait and poor balance.

> I had heard that one way of dealing with this change was to go on an imaginary journey to a harbour of acceptance and to stand on the harbour wall and formally say goodbye to whatever it was that you had lost, that way you could start to come to terms with that loss. I can remember the instant well because I was travelling back to Newcastle on the train from London and so had nothing else to do. I closed my eyes and imagined my legs doing all the things I used to value and enjoy and then boarded those images onto the ship waiting at the quayside. I then sat and watched it sail away taking those images with it. All this probably sounds really weird but it really did help to have once and for all have said goodbye and to stop struggling to hang on to something I knew I had lost. That doesn't mean that I don't still miss them but at the time I think it helped.

It is difficult to convey such feelings in clinical terms but hopefully the experiences of some of the clients quoted can convey the intensity of emotion clients are having to cope with in relation to adjusting to a new image of themselves, the way they look to other people and the way in which their body functions. This adjustment of self-image is not, for clients with rheumatoid disease, a one-off adjustment as over a period of ten years many different adjustments may have to be made as the disease progresses.

As professionals it is easy to sit back and state that society is becoming more aware of the needs of people with disabilities and integration is really beginning to happen, but a frank discussion with many clients will emphasize how much further we have to go. Many instances can be given of clients having to confront prejudice and curiosity ranging from 'By you're a bit of a cripple aren't you pet?' to 'What's someone like you doing in a thing like that?' (a wheelchair.)

Therapists may feel that there is little they can do to help but the abilities to listen, to support and to show empathy can go a long way to helping clients express this loss and start to adjust to change. A frequently used opening line is 'I know you will think that I am vain but . . .' Whether considered vain or not, self-image is a highly valued component of self-concept and the loss associated with it is as great as the loss associated with any other component of self-concept or facet of function and should be acknowledged as such.

CHANGES IN ROLE

Role is a way of describing the various relationships that a person perceives themselves to have with society or another person. They may be related to work, social or family settings. Social roles are used to identify an organized pattern of behaviour that is characteristic and expected of the occupant of a defined position in a social system, Mosey (1986). Most people are adopting several roles at any one time, e.g. worker, friend, parent, sister and daughter.

A role exists in relation to a role partner, i.e. husband–wife, mother–daughter and as well as having a partner, comprises a task behaviour and an interpersonal behaviour. The task behaviour refers to the activities encompassed in the role and the interpersonal behaviour relates to the interactions that are required while fulfilling the role.

The onset of a chronic disease can often threaten a client's ability to maintain existing roles and in some cases necessitate the adoption of new ones. Limitation in functional activities may compromise a client's ability to carry out tasks required to fulfil the role and interpersonal behaviours may change due to the response of the client or other role participants to the development of a disability or handicap. This section will examine how a chronic disease can affect the role within the work setting, the family environment and the community as a whole.

Roles related to employment

Work roles become incorporated into self-image during the late teens and early twenties when work becomes a part of daily life for most people. Work provides a structure and routine to the day, a challenge in terms of planning a career and providing goals to aim for, a sense of contributing to society and a certain amount of financial security.

Clients with rheumatoid disease have to face many challenges within the work environment. Morning stiffness and the extra time needed to complete tasks can mean the day has to begin much earlier in order to be at work on time. The variability in the disease can lead to inconsistent levels of performance, not only from day to day but also throughout the day, and periods of exacerbation can lead to extended time away from work, as can periods of hospital admission.

The healthcare system does not function in a way that assists clients in employment. As clinics are held mainly during the working day, time off work may be required frequently. A client prescribed a course of gold therapy is required to make frequent and sometimes lengthy trips to the hospital, perhaps stretching the goodwill of some employers and placing pressure on the client who may be all too aware of possible criticism. The same is true for other therapeutic interventions which the client may be in need of and may be a cause of the client not attending. Clients will inevitably be placed in the position of determining the most valuable appointments to attend and those which may be useful but not necessary.

The attitudes of colleagues and employers play a central role in a person being able to maintain their work and cope with their changing needs. Fear of dismissal, in an age of high unemployment, may lead clients to try to conceal their problems for as long as possible. To some extent the ability to maintain a job is dependent upon the employer's response to the needs of their employees. A flexible approach to problem solving and an acknowledgement of an employee's potential rather than limitations can lead to functional problems being overcome. While physical barriers are often surmountable social barriers are more difficult to overcome.

Clients who are unemployed and seeking employment often have to over-come both physical barriers and social stereotypes of the abilities and disabilities of a person with a handicap. Clients find that prejudice and lack of understanding lead frequently to applications being turned down without interview if they declare a disability.

Clients seeking further education or training are faced often with physical barriers of inaccessible colleges or training centres and in many cases job centres, placing them at a huge disadvantage. If buildings are accessible specialist equipment is often not available to enable clients to participate fully in all courses. If the client's degree of handicap is such that they need assistance with personal care then their ability to participate is reduced even more.

A situation encountered by many younger people seeking advice regarding careers or changes in career is that professionals have narrow concepts of careers which may be pursued, often they are pointed in the direction of clerical or administrative work.

Two factors have been identified as decreasing the probability of having to leave work due to disability, first, a substantial degree of work place autonomy, and second, self-employment (Meenan et al., 1981). In both of these situations the client is in a position to control their working environment and adapt it to suit their needs.

Maintaining a job can lead to compromises in other aspects of a client's life, especially in relation to leisure and social activities. The energy required to complete a full day's work may dictate that evenings and weekends are spent resting. Although, in the short term, this may resolve an immediate need, which is to remain in employment, in the long term it can lead to a decrease in social contacts. While in employment the loss of social contacts may not appear too important, as work itself will provide alternatives. But if a person is forced to give up work their social network will be rapidly reduced and isolation may occur.

The decision to leave work for many clients highlights a time of stress. It is unusual if this decision is taken and acted upon instantaneously, for many clients it usually follows a prolonged period of being away from work and a gradual awareness that return to work is not a realistic aim. This period of time can necessitate a reappraisal of self-concept and role, as the identity of worker may no longer be one of the main roles associated with self. Ceasing employment can also be equated with an apparent deterioration in functional ability. In Meenan's study of 245 people with rheumatoid disease, 59% of those who had jobs no longer worked and of those, 89% attributed this to their rheumatoid disease. For those people their earning potential was reduced by 50% (Meenan et al., 1981).

The value of work to people is high, especially in an age of high unemployment. Most people who become unemployed can ascribe the loss of work to a factor external to themselves and beyond their control, such as government policy or the economic climate. The focusing of blame on an external factor does not require that the individual has to come to terms with the fact that a deterioration in their own functional ability has led to them having to give up work. For clients leaving work due to their rheumatoid disease a double loss is incurred, first the role of worker and second the loss of functional ability.

The losses related to this period of time are immense and include

25

change in role, financial loss, and a loss of structure and purpose to the day. The financial loss may not only be associated with a change in standard of living but may also be a time of transition from financial independence to dependence upon the State.

The change in role is every bit as pertinent to the housewife who is no longer able to carry out her function within the home. In some ways this change is even harder to cope with as she is confronted daily by her inability to complete tasks. This frustration is often compounded by having to watch someone else carry out the work, often in a different way and to a different standard or else having to ask another family member to help. The introduction of a home help, a matter of routine for many professionals, represents a confrontation with a loss of role for the housewife.

If the role of worker is no longer seen as a component of identity the value ascribed to this role is reassessed. Other roles may be given a higher value to make up for the loss, and so a role within the family may become more important or new roles may be adopted, a client may begin on a course of further education for example. High levels of energy and motivation are required to identify potential resources and explore the possibilities of alternative roles at a time when fatigue, pain and limitations in functional ability have led to employment having to be given up. This can limit the exploration of alternatives. Other limitations on the adoption of new roles may be the change in a client's financial status, a degree of expense is usually incurred by most forms of hobby, educational or recreational pursuit, or the physical barriers of access to buildings or the availability of specialist equipment. While many excellent opportunities now exist for study at home, via the Open University or Open College, these options do not overcome the social isolation often experienced on ceasing employment.

Role within the family environment

The onset of a chronic disease in one member of a family unit will inevitably affect the whole unit. The term 'handicapped family' has been used to described this concept (Shearer, 1981). This can apply to both the immediate and extended family.

The status of the handicapped person within the family may change in many ways, from breadwinner to dependent, from the dominant partner to a more passive role and from a position of independence to one of dependence. If one member of the family adopts a new role the role of the other family members may have to alter to accommodate this change. If role reversal occurs, i.e. the dominant partner is required to become more passive and the passive partner is required to become more dominant, stress and anxiety can be felt by both partners especially if the new role to be adopted is one in which neither person feels happy or wishes to adopt. The dynamics of the family will have been altered.

Many roles are socially defined and carry with them a set of attributes and functions which are perceived as being necessary to fulfil in order to maintain the role. One example of this is the way in which the role of 'mother' can be threatened for many women. After giving birth some women experience a period of increased disease activity and consequently experience difficulty in caring for the newly born baby. Feeding, changing and even holding the baby can be difficult. The emotional turmoil associated with childbirth can be exacerbated by the inability to care for the baby, in the expected way, and a dependence upon another family member. If the children are older they may be required to assist with tasks around the house or in some situations help with more personal activities such as bathing or dressing. This may lead a parent to feel guilt as the children are being asked to give up time which for them may otherwise have been spent playing or studying and has been expressed as 'denying them their childhood'. These intense emotions associated with a perceived 'failure' as a parent are often encountered during discussions. The feeling of guilt is another emotion expressed frequently in relation to the way families are often the recipients of bad tempers when clients feel frustrated or in pain.

Isolation can be experienced within the family for a number of reasons. Pain or sleepless nights may lead to partners sleeping in separate beds or separate rooms, fatigue or lack of energy may lead to the client sleeping during the day or in the evening and not going out as a member of a family so often. Physical isolation can be experienced through a lessening of physical contact due to increased pain making hugging painful or fear on the families' behalf of causing pain. Decreased mobility can mean that clients may not be able to join in all the family activities possibly staying at home on some occasions.

The needs of partners are not always given as much consideration as they should be, the focus being primarily upon the client. Misconceptions about the disease can make understanding what is happening to the client difficult. Anger, resentment and frustration are also experienced by partners as their plans, hopes for the future and lifestyle will be affected as much as the clients. The expression of these emotions can be difficult for partners. 'How can you verbalize negative feelings about a situation which is beyond your control, especially when you are daily having to watch your partner struggle and cope with pain? Who do you share these feelings with who will understand and not think you are being selfish?' Partners can feel that they are betraying their partner by voicing difficulties to other people or may feel that they themselves will be seen as unsupportive and uncaring. The inability to voice these feelings can lead to stress within a relationship.

Partners are also confronted with the guilt associated with carrying out activities alone which were previously carried out together, or going out with the family and leaving the partner at home. One husband expressed how if he went out alone and had a good time he had to live down his enjoyment when he returned home to his wife as she had had to stay at home alone. This guilt is often expressed by partners who are caring for a highly-dependent client who may be taken into hospital for a period of respite care. Partners can see this as a reflection of their inability to cope or as letting their partner down and may find it difficult to use the time as it was meant, i.e. to have a rest and to take some time for themselves. A frequent experience of caring agencies in this situation is that the client's partner spends most of the week travelling to visit the client in hospital.

The social isolation which can be experienced by a client can also be experienced by their husbands or wives, especially if the client is limited in their functional ability. Many therapists will have been in contact with families where their whole lives revolve around completing the essential activities of daily living and coping with the number of professionals calling to assist them. The carer's life can become very limited with little or no time for hobbies or social activities. Carers in this situation often relate how, when their partner has been taken into long-term care or has died, they have had to completely rebuild their life again as their circle of friends has diminished and they had in many ways ceased to exist as a person in their own right. Partners are required to redefine their role and relationship as well as the client.

The attitude of the carer towards illness and disability can also influence the client's behaviour. Carers can be protective taking-over many of the functional activities from the client because they do not know when to stand back and watch their partner struggle and when to step in and help. The reality of family life may mean that it is quicker for partners to do things themselves, especially first thing in the morning. Alternatively some partners are unable to come to terms with the changes occurring and try to cope by ignoring the fact that anything has changed and expect life to continue as before, making few, if any, concessions to the pain and difficulties their partner may be experiencing.

The involvement of other family members is essential in the management of rheumatoid disease. They are the people who are required to provide support and motivation and who also have their own needs in coming to terms with the affect upon their life and future. Their roles will be significantly altered, future plans affected and feelings of frustration, anger and stress encountered alongside those of their partners. They have even less control than the client over changes which may be occurring due to the disease and are placed therefore in an even more passive role.

Role within the community

The way in which a society responds to people with disabilities can affect dramatically the way in which people can function within that society and the roles which they can adopt. Societies can build both physical and psychological barriers which prevent full integration. The general public's concept of a person with a disability is generally a negative one providing a huge barrier which has to be overcome on numerous occasions. The word 'disabled' is negative, being ascribed such definitions as, 'to deprive of power, to weaken, to cripple, and to deprecate' (Hayward and Sparks, 1986).

It is argued that it is in fact society that is handicapped by its understanding of handicap and that the boundaries of normality should be widened as every member of society has inabilities which will to some degree handicap the way in which they function (Shearer, 1981).

Cultural factors will also affect the way in which a person's role may change if they become disabled. In some eastern cultures the person is cared for totally within the family environment and the need for that person to become independent is not perceived, where as in some western societies people with disabilities fight vociferously for their right to function independently within society and for that society to recognize that right and where necessary adapt to meet it. Cultural influences become more important to therapists who are now working in multi-racial communities where roles, expectations and outcomes can vary enormously between cultures and therapists should have an appreciation of such differences.

The society in which we have been brought up will shape our attitudes towards people with disabilities and these attitudes will affect the way in which we perceive ourselves should we ever develop a disability. A person who perceives people with disabilities as weak, having little to offer and as an object of pity may experience difficulty equating that concept to themselves if they should develop a disability. People's concept of 'disabled people' may be why clients will do all that they can to avoid being called disabled. Therapists are often told by clients 'you can always look around and see someone who is worse off' perhaps this is a way of seeking reassurance that a certain stage perceived as 'disabled' has not yet been reached.

The fear of being stigmatized brings with it an unspoken pressure for some people of needing to achieve a higher level of success and attainment in order to prove that a disabled person can cope as well as, if not better than, anyone else.

The physical environment also provides daily challenges to integration within society ranging from negotiating public transport systems to gaining access to public buildings. Feelings of vulnerability and insecurity within this threatening environment can be a cause of isolation and withdrawal. An observation made by many clients is the lack of seating within shops and department stores if a rest is required. Walking in busy streets can be frightening if balance is not very good or lower limbs are apt to 'give way'. Activities which were previously carried out with little thought can become so complicated that the effort involved becomes prohibitive. For a person with limited mobility the spontaneity of going to, for example, the theatre is taken away. If you need to use a wheelchair you may have to inform the theatre of your intention of going so that arrangements can be made to get you in and once inside you are given little option of where you can sit, and the bar and toilets are very likely inaccessible to you.

The barriers to the integration of people with disabilities into society are immense and erected throughout the whole strata of society from the individual, to the statutory sector, local and central government. Overcoming these barriers is an ongoing problem which occurs every time a person with a disability enters that society and therefore the energy and physical ability required is often not available to that person and the effort is wearing. As a disease progresses and function deteriorates the effort increases and one way of coping with this situation is to withdraw from such confrontations or to cease responding and fighting. By doing this people's social environment can become smaller and they can become the passive recipient of societies' prejudices. While it is often said that people with disabilities are discriminated against no more than any other minority group and their predicament is similar it must be remembered that while this may be true, coping with and confronting prejudice is more difficult when you cannot physically gain access to buildings, when functional ability may be limited and when energy may be depleted. The extension of a disability into a handicap is often the result of societal attitudes, values and the handicapping environment in which we exist.

The role of patient

While aspects of other roles are being lost due to the onset of a chronic disease one which is being assimilated into self-concept is that of patient. This role will have different connotations for different people but is usually equated with being 'sick' and in need of treatment. The role of patient is reinforced by the environment in which that role is encountered, i.e. hospitals and doctors' surgeries and the perceived roles of the people working within that environment. The environment encountered in many hospitals is rigid, authoritarian and oppressive and is primarily equipped to deal with acute illness. When an individual comes into contact with such an environment it is difficult to adopt anything other than a passive role. In relation to acute illness this may be appropriate as many patients are not in a position to participate in what is happening to them. However, the situation changes in relation to a chronic disease when clients are not in a life-threatening situation.

A classical example of this, in this country, is the way in which client's medication is taken away from them as soon as they walk through the door of a ward. The client has probably been managing, very successfully, to administer their own medication for the last five years, but simply by virtue of walking through a doorway is no longer responsible enough to carry on so doing. Some units have realized the irrationality behind this and have had to fight extremely hard to overcome the rigidity of rules governing the administration of medication. Self-medication on some wards has now been achieved, but these are still very much in the minority.

Many such examples can be given of ways in which hospital environments and the attitudes of people working within those environments can become oppressive and this is an important factor which is especially pertinent when considering the role which clients are to take in the management of their disease. Is it appropriate, or indeed possible to try and promote self-management programmes and active roles in an environment which reinforces passivity and reliance upon 'professionals' and how many divergent messages are clients receiving?

The expectations of many clients coming into contact with healthcare professionals is that they will identify the problem and prescribe a treatment which will eliminate or alleviate the cause. Clients are, therefore, being asked to alter their expectations of healthcare professionals and accept a degree of responsibility for their own healthcare. It can be argued that the advent of the National Health Service changed the emphasis of responsibility for health. People began to look to the NHS for their health needs when previously they had dealt with many of their own problems.

STAGES IN LIFE

The most common time of disease onset is between the ages of thirty and fifty. To begin to understand the impact of a chronic disease it is necessary to consider some of the general issues which are being addressed during these periods of life and may be effected by the onset of a disease.

Early adulthood 20–35

This is the time during which independence from parents usually occurs, both physically and psychologically. Decisions are also taken regarding career and personal relationships. The role of worker becomes established into self-concept and alongside this financial independence is achieved from parents. With regard to personal relationships the main issues which are addressed relate to the conflict between finding a partner and settling into a permanent relationship or remaining single and uncommitted to any one person. Once a commitment has been made decisions are then faced regarding becoming a parent.

For a person developing rheumatoid disease during this period all of these aspects can become threatened. A single person may question their ability to form and sustain a personal relationship and question their attractiveness. They may worry about how deterioration in years to come may make them dependent upon their partner and the legitimacy of knowingly burdening someone else with their problems. Opposition from prospective in-laws may be encountered. Clients in a stable personal relationship may have to confront the possible changes which take place within that relationship and how their partner feels about those changes. This may involve changes in plans to start a family, or possibly changes in financial status may limit the previous standard of living.

If the client is still living at home with their parents achieving independence may become more difficult, both physically and psychologically. For some clients this independence may already have been achieved but limitations in functional ability or constraints on income due to having to cease employment may lead to having to move back into the parental home and increased dependence. This can be seen as a retrigrade step and will inevitably effect the lives of the client and their family.

In terms of career gaining employment may be difficult as employers may not feel happy taking on an employee with a chronic disease and need convincing that the contribution that can be made will outweigh any possible physical limitations the person may have. Long term career plans may change in the light of possible functional limitations and perceived prospects may alter. The ability to carry out full time employment is compromised often by the variable nature of the disease and the functional limitations occurring as a result of pain, stiffness and loss of movement.

Middle adulthood 35–60

This is usually the age group which is running society in terms of responsibility and power. Careers have usually progressed and positions of responsibility have been achieved. Families are growing up and leaving home. Coping with adolescent children presents many challenges and also represents a time at which the family is becoming less dependent upon parents. This can lead to a period of reassessment and questions related to how the role of parent will change and what other role may be adopted to accommodate this change. As one's own parents are approaching old age this period may also include an increasing need to care for them.

This period represents the most common age of disease onset and therefore is the age group most frequently encountered in a rheumatology department. Development of a chronic disease during this period can require a reassessment of role in relation to work, family and society. The prospect of having to give up work can be devastating, especially as the position reached may represent years of work. Anger and resentment can be directed towards the fact that, especially towards the end of this period, children are becoming less dependent and plans may have been directed towards spending more time with partners and planning for retirement. These plans may have to change considerably.

Post-retirement 60 onwards

Clients during this period of their life may be having to face a change in role as they or their partner reaches retirement age, the assimilation of role as grandparent into their self-concept and an increasing dependency upon the state and their family. When retired, partners are able to spend more time together, developing social and leisure activities. If a client is married they may have to cope with the death of their partner and have to consider how functional problems can be overcome alone. While for some clients this may mean increased dependence upon homecare services, their family or moving into sheltered or residential homes, for others it can lead to an increase in functional ability. One client began to do more for herself after the death of her husband than she had done for a long time, her independence increased significantly.

The development of a chronic disease, during any stage in life, can lead to a period of reassessment and re-evaluation of self-concept. As this is not self-imposed varying amounts of stress and anxiety will be experienced.

STRESS ANXIETY AND DEPRESSION

The experience of stress is an emotional one and is therefore a totally unique experience, expressed in emotional and subjective terms. A situation which is perceived as stressful by one person may not be by another. A transactional model of stress has been proposed by Cox and Mackay which defines stress as 'a perceptual phenomenon arising between the demand on a person and his ability to cope. An imbalance in this mechanism when coping is important giving rise to the experience of stress and the stress response' (Cox, 1978). The response to stress depends upon how a person perceives the demand confronting them and their ability to cope. This process starts with an appraisal of the situation which initially defines the meaning of the stress and whether it entails a threat, a challenge or actual harm and then progresses to identifying ways in which the stress can be dealt with.

Dealing with stress depends upon past experience and the resources and skills available to the person and requires the use of coping strategies. Therefore, a level of stress is necessary to elicit the use of coping strategies but it is the discrepancy between what each individual perceives to be the demands being made upon them and the strategies available to them that can lead to anxiety, depression and feelings of helplessness.

Feeling out of control can lead to high levels of stress. This can be induced by the variability and unpredictability of the disease process or entering a system of care which is unfamiliar and therefore increases reliance upon other people. Changes in self-concept, especially when forced upon a person also leads to stress and anxiety. Many of the situations confronting a client with rheumatoid disease will be potentially stressful and anxiety provoking. Consideration should be given to ways in which this stress can be reduced to manageable levels and clients helped to develop some of the skills to cope effectively with stressful situations regaining some degree of control and lessening stress.

Consideration should also be given to ways in which clients can be helped to minimize or deal with symptoms of stress by the use of techniques such as relaxation, biofeedback or counselling. It is unusual for stress to reach such levels that acute anxiety states are reached and medical intervention needed, but this will depend upon a client's previous personality and how they dealt with stress prior to the onset of rheumatoid disease.

Reviews of literature will introduce the concept of an 'arthritic personality' which is based upon personality traits which predispose a client to the onset of rheumatoid disease. This concept is associated with mainly negative personality traits such as conforming, inhibited and lacking in emotional expression. Several reviews of this literature have been carried out and have identified flaws in both the design methods and evaluative procedures. In his review of psychological aspects of rheumatoid disease Baum found that from 100 studies published 'more than 50% of the studies used psychological tests that were devised by the investigator and not used by any other group' (Baum, 1982). The main criticisms of these studies have been those relating to lack of controls, validity, and reliability of measures and the retrospective nature of the studies. Anderson concludes 'there is little or no support for the existence of an arthritis personality that predates the disease and in some way leads to the disease onset. Negative personality characteristics are more feasibly explained as reactions to this chronic disease rather than a causal factor' (Anderson *et al.*, 1985).

However, an area undergoing research is that of the relationship of psychological factors and disease activity, especially the effects of stress. Subjective discussions with clients will often highlight stress as a cause of an exacerbation in disease activity, and in some instances as a cause of the disease. In a study carried out by Rimon two specific sub-groups were identified, a major conflict group characterized by little or no family history of rheumatoid disease, severe symptoms and sudden onset, and a non-conflict group, where there was a higher hereditary predisposition, onset was insiduous and disease progress was slow. The major conflict group were able to identify an emotionally traumatic life event within a year before disease onset and associated subsequent flares with emotional trauma (Rimon, 1985).

These observations were, however, based upon non-directed interviews and could be explained by the process of attribution in which a client is seeking a causal factor to initiate the disease onset. It could also be that increased disease activity lowers a client's ability to cope and as a result of decreased coping higher levels of stress are experienced. When discussing the relationship of stress to disease activity the distinction has not as yet been made between a causal factor or a response and is an area of ongoing research.

The occurrence of depression as a response to chronic illness should be seen as a normal response and not one necessarily requiring pharmaceutical intervention, unless it reaches the stages of clinical depression or impairs a client's function. A reactive depression to loss of function, changes in self-concept and coping with chronic pain is frequently encountered in clients at some stage in the course of their disease. The opportunity to discuss these feelings and to be given support and counselling should be available to clients as they often feel that their family has reached the point of overload and they can no longer 'burden them with their problems' so the availability of another person with whom to express and explore their feelings is often helpful. This does not necessarily have to be a member of a clinical team and may just as well be a friend, but for some clients limited function and mobility can limit access to friends or other resources which they may previously have used to work through depressive feelings prior to disease onset.

To deal with the emotions of stress, anxiety and depression a client is required to utilize a variety of different coping strategies.

Coping strategies

A coping strategy can be defined as 'any thought or action which succeeds in eliminating or ameliorating threat . . . whether it is consciously recognized as intentional or not' (Breakwell, 1986). The range of coping strategies used will differ from person to person and situation to situation. The failure of one strategy to deal with the threat may lead to the use of another. Three levels of coping strategies have been identified by Breakwell:

1. intrapsychic, involving emotions and cognitions;
2. interpersonal, relying on changing relationships with others;
3. intergroup, which directs threat at the individual as a member of a group lessening the impact.

Intrapsychic strategies include such techniques as selective ignoring, denial and the modification of self-concept. The use of selective ignoral and denial aims to deflect the threat, 'this is not really happening to me', 'it will go away as quickly as it came'. Techniques which aim to accept the threat include modifying self-concept, one method of doing this is to re-evaluate aspects of self-concept by devaluing an activity or role which can no longer be carried out or placing a higher value on another activity to take its place.

Interpersonal strategies are aimed at modifying relationships with others. Two such strategies pertinent to rheumatology are those of isolation and compliance. If a person feels threatened in a situation one way of dealing with it is to withdraw from the situation and avoid placing oneself in that situation again. This does not deal with the stress but removes the necessity to confront it.

This strategy is encountered as a way in which clients deal with peoples responses to deformity and also in coping with situations which may highlight areas of limitation. While this strategy may be a way of coping with one form of stress it can often bring about another one, that of coping with the subsequent isolation that can follow as a consequence.

The concept of compliance is difficult to address as its meaning varies according to the context in which it is used. A therapist may on the one hand be working to increase a client's compliance with an exercise programme, but, on the other hand be trying to decrease their compliance to the 'sick role'. If a client adopts a compliant role and is continually placed in a position of passivity they will eventually learn passivity and become 'helpless' in decision making, losing previous skills and becoming dependent.

Intergroup coping strategies are aimed at lessening the impact of the disease on the individual by facilitating self-help, providing a supportive environment and undertaking specific action in the form of pressure groups.

With a variety of coping strategies available a person may choose one or a combination of strategies to deal with a specific problem. In his work related to the management of illness Mechanic identified a 'search for meaning' (Mechanic, 1977) as a prerequisite for coping. He maintained that it was only through an understanding of what is happening that reasonable response could be devised.

The identification of a causal factor related to rheumatoid disease has not been found. Gaining a sense of understanding can be difficult in relation to a disease where there is no apparent causal factor, fluctuation in disease activity has no apparent cause and answers to questions are usually generalized, vague or evasive.

LOCUS OF CONTROL

The amount of control a person feels they have in the management of their condition will effect their response to the disease, the treatment they utilize and the coping strategies they use. Locus of control is a concept which describes this process and represents a continuum from internal to external. A person with an internal locus of control feels that they have some degree of influence over their disease and takes on some of the responsibility for its management. A person with an external locus of control feels that their disease is beyond their influence and tends to adopt a passive role in its management negating responsibility for what is occurring.

A client taking on a degree of control is acknowledging their influence and responsibility in the disease management. In the course of the disease there will inevitably be periods of fluctuation in levels of function and pain. A person with an internal locus of control may feel responsible for this change and ascribe it to failure on their own behalf leading to a sense of no longer having control and helplessness. This feeling of losing control can lead to high levels of stress and anxiety. It is at this time that therapists who work towards increasing clients control should provide support and counselling to help clients regain feelings of control. A person with an external locus of control will ascribe such changes to factors other than their own limitations which acts as a form of defence strategy.

The unpredictable nature of rheumatoid disease adds to the difficulty of feeling in control. An increase in disease activity can occur for no apparent reason and without warning, making forward planning difficult. Arrangements, therefore, need to be kept fluid to accommodate any change in condition. This includes social activities, holidays and other events which would previously have been planned in advance and anticipated with pleasure.

The resources used in coping are varied and have been categorized by Pearlin and Schooler as social, psychological, and specific coping responses (Pearlin and Schooler, 1978). Social resources relate to family, friends, colleagues etc., psychological resources relate to personality characteristics and specific coping responses relates to the behaviours, cognitions and perceptions engaged in to deal with a problem. These resources are inter-related and affect each other. Mechanic (1977) has addressed the issue of social adaptation to illness and identified several factors affecting adaptation. These are,

1. economic resources, largely influenced by government policy;
2. the abilities and skills of the individual;
3. defensive techniques;
4. social support;
5. motivation.

He suggests that 'the adequacy of any individual to cope depends on the effectiveness of cultural preparation and the availability of problem-solving tools necessary to deal with typical problems. What may be an ordinary situation for those with skills or adequate preparation is a crisis for those who lack them'. Many clients will be encountering new situations and problems and may not necessarily have developed ways of dealing with them. The strategies used and developed will vary considerably and change as new situations are encountered. Previously-used strategies may no longer be effective and so clients need access to a range of skills to enable them to cope with the diverse situations they will inevitably encounter.

This chapter has hopefully provided an insight into some of the psychosocial problems which can be encountered by clients. The psychosocial effects of a chronic disease can be phenomenal, requiring fundamental changes in self-concept, threatening previously held identities and having as profound an effect as the physical manifestations of the disease on the way in which a person functions. It is essential for therapists and clinicians to gain an understanding of these processes if they are to assist, in any meaningful way, clients to adapt to living with rheumatoid disease.

FURTHER READING

G. Breakwell (1986) *Coping with Threatened Identities*, Methuen.

T. Cox (1987) *Stress* Macmillan Education, London.

V. Finkelstein (1980) *Attitudes and Disabled People*, World Rehabilitation Fund.

D. Locker (1983) *Disability and Disadvantage. The Consequences of Chronic Illness*, Tavistock Publications Ltd, London.

A. Shearer (1981) *Disability Whose Handicap*, Blackwell, Oxford.

3

An holistic approach to the management of rheumatoid disease

The two previous chapters have outlined the complexity of rheumatoid disease in relation to its physical, psychological and social manifestations. The relationship between these different dimensions is totally unique to each individual client and also variable, for the individual, throughout the course of the disease, therefore posing a challenge to clinical management. The range of needs which may be expressed by one client requires a variety of treatment strategies to be available and the lack of knowledge about the disease and effectiveness of interventions necessitates a broad programme of clinical and laboratory-based research to be undertaken. No single treatment technique has, as yet, been identified as having a major impact on the disease process and its manifestations, therefore clinical management still remains multi-faceted and primarily aimed at coping with the effects of the disease.

This is seen in the multi-disciplinary approach used in most rheumatology departments which encompasses laboratory work, directed at understanding the mechanism of the disease,clinical research, directed towards evaluating the effectiveness of different forms of intervention, and the clinical management of the physical, psychological and social problems presented by individual clients.

This team approach, when working well, has the potential to offer a range of treatment techniques and the opportunities for clients to explore a variety of possible coping strategies. These range from directed self-management courses, providing practical information, to non-directed group work, providing an environment in which clients can explore and identify their own needs in coping with a chronic disease, from pharmaceutical methods of pain control to relaxation techniques and from specific treatment programmes to the development of skills related to activities such as art, literature and music.

The potential of the team is dependent largely upon its members' concept and definition of its composites and their understanding of the potential skills of each other. If the concept is rigid and limited to a few people the potential is limited and clients will only have direct access to resources which lie within this boundary. A lack of understanding of each others' skills and resources leads to an under-utilization of the team's potential. Frequently, in clinical practice, the needs of an individual are met as long as they fall within the constraints of a 'team', thus limiting the range of options available.

Clients are referred to dieticians for advice on weight-reducing diets but few have access routinely to dieticians for advice if they wish to explore the possibility of using diet as a means of controlling their disease activity. A high percentage of clients will at some time try a different diet and need access to information on basic nutrition and ways of ensuring a balanced diet. Dieticians have the relevant skills and information but bias against this strategy as a component of management denies clients access to information and forces them to look to libraries, or private practitioners for advice.

Pain control clinics are used frequently for clients with chronic pain, usually which has not been amenable to pharmaceutical methods of control, and a range of methods of pain control are explored, both pharmaceutical and non-pharmaceutical. These alternative methods of controlling pain are not available widely to the main population of a rheumatology department despite pain being the main reason for referral and client's, and clinician's, unhappiness with the long-term effects of taking nonsteroidal anti-inflammatory medication.

The above examples relate to resources which are already a component of healthcare within the statutory sector but which possibly have the potential to add to the strategies available to clients and clinicians in coping with rheumatoid disease. The role of social sciences, art and religion are often perceived as lying outside the remit of a team, alongside alternative medicine, although all are frequently turned to by clients as a way of coping with certain problems. Their contribution and validity is questioned by clinicians.

The need to establish the validity of approaches is central to the medical model of care to ensure that, as a minimum requirement, the potential to do harm is eliminated. Inclusion within this medical framework is dependent upon meeting these criteria. Establishing the validity of an approach by ascribing numerical values to concepts with high degrees of variability is fraught with difficulty and has to a large degree been avoided.

While this situation remains static a continuous argument exists in which potentially valuable components of management are being discounted and clients are forced to look outside the recognized system for help. The onus has to be upon practitioners to validate the interventions they are using but the open-mindedness of clinicians to explore beyond a rigid definition of a team may assist in establishing the validity of alternative forms of intervention. A reappraisal of potential resources which are deemed frequently to be on the periphery of care may open a wider range of options to clients which are more appropriate in addressing the wide range of needs of the clients.

The potential number of people involved in the treatment and support of a client with rheumatoid disease is large, involving hospital and community based services from the statutory and voluntary sectors. The involvement of agencies will depend upon the needs of each client with some requiring relatively few and others needing many. The communication of information between services can be a problem which increases in direct proportion to the number of services involved. The availability and communication of information is a key element in the planning and implementation of an effective treatment programme. The identification of a key worker to liaise between agencies, especially between hospital and community services is essential to ensure continuity of approach.

THE RELATIONSHIP OF MULTI-DISCIPLINARY TEAMS AND CLIENTS

The effective functioning of a team is also dependent upon the role the client is asked to adopt within this team. They are the one person who will be in contact with all the agencies involved in their management, which in relation to the rest of the team is a unique position. If they have been active in the planning of their treatment and understand the basis of decisions which have been made they can be central to the functioning of a team approach. If they have no involvement at all they then become a pawn moved through a variety of experiences without understanding why or being able to contribute in any way other than that of passive recipient. A cynic may say that this is the most efficient way to run a team which is professionally led.

Many therapists will have been confronted with clients arriving in the department not knowing why they have been referred, sometimes even who has referred them, or what is going to happen to them when they arrive. As professionals it is all too easy to adopt the 'I did explain' approach which usually means that at some point during a consultation an explanation was given but the client did not understand. An awareness must develop, amongst professionals, of the feelings experienced by clients when placed in a clinical environment over which they have little control and at a time when their stress levels are high. The onus should be placed upon the professional to create an environment which is less intimidating, ensure that information is communicated and to check that this has been understood.

Consideration should also be given to which team member will be the most effective in communicating information. After a ward round has passed through a ward more information is usually communicated to clients from nurses returning to talk than at the time the round has reached the client's bed. Clients can feel so anxious by the presence of so many people and of being the focus of attention that they are unable to assimilate what is being said. While communicating information may be a time consuming process it is essential if the client is to function as a member of the team.

Access to information and potential resources is to a large degree controlled by 'professionals' and their perception of what clients need to know. If the knowledge of the team regarding the resources available is limited this limitation will be passed on to the client. While it can be argued that the client has the option to find out information for themselves the time, functional ability, energy, and skills needed to do so are not always present. The barriers to gaining information are numerous, ranging from the ways in which professionals can discourage and limit self-help to the format of the information once it is identified. As a result of the 1986 Disabled Persons Act, Local Authorities now have a statutory obligation to provide information on the services which they provide to clients. No such statute, as yet, applies to Health Authorities and clients rarely know how they gain access to dieticians, chiropodists, appliance officers etc. The same applies to the voluntary sector which is often more confusing and so clients remain reliant upon clinicians to raise their awareness of resources which can be used.

The nature of rheumatoid disease necessitates a team approach to management which is holistic in nature. The needs of the individual have to be the focus of the clinical team not solely the disease, as the physical, psychological, social and spiritual make-up of the individual will determine the way in which they experience and respond to the disease.

While the central role of the client in their treatment programme is discussed frequently the implementation of such an approach and the definition of what that role entails is an extremely grey area. In many cases it entails explaining the rationale of interventions to clients as they are about to happen or providing information about areas of assumed interest. The use of a truly client-directed approach would change the basis of much clinical practice, if implemented, and require a great deal of energy, time and resources from all team members, including clients themselves. There are many barriers which have to be overcome for this to be a reality and many areas of conflict to address. Some of these issues will be raised in subsequent chapters and cover the whole spectrum of physical, social and psychological barriers for both client and practitioner. The composites of the team are varied and can include any of the following.

1. Hospital based team:
   Consultant
   Surgeon;
   Nurse;
   Occupational therapist;
   Physiotherapist;
   Social worker;
   Psychologist;
   Pharmacist;
   Dietician;
   Orthotist;
   Chiropodist.
2. Community based team:
   General practitioner;
   District nurse;
   Occupational therapist;
   Support Services, home help, meals on wheels, bath attendant;
   Employment Agencies;
   Housing department.
3. Non Statutory Agencies:
   Voluntary organizations;
   Church;
   Complementary medicine.
4. Research team:
   Laboratory team;
   Clinical team comprising any of the above.

This list is by no means exhaustive but provides an indication of the complexity of co-ordinating and evaluating appropriate interventions. The availability of the above resources will vary and will be influenced by some extent to economic, social and political factors.

Economic factors

Certainly within the statutory sector economic factors are becoming one of the major influences on service provision and the delivery of health care. The perceived cost of providing institutional care has led to a shift in emphasis to community care which has not necessarily seen the transfer of resources to accommodate this change. The change in emphasis has to some extent highlighted areas of concern regarding the ability of community services within the statutory sector to cope with this change. In addition the role of the voluntary sector is changing as greater demands are being placed upon it and it is now becoming an integral component of healthcare in relation to chronic disability.

However, the major effect of economic factors on therapists is that the need to evaluate the effectiveness of intervention is becoming more widely recognized in order to compete for resources. The development of performance indicators and cost benefit analysis is going to mean that, for the first time, therapists will need to be able to justify some of their treatment and interventions. Budget holders will want to know the value of what they are paying for and blanket referrals will probably disappear.

With increasing case loads and, in the community, growing waiting lists, the need to consider carefully the allocation of resources and the establishment of priorities for the service appears. Given a 36 hour week and an expanding case load decisions are having to be made as to the most effective way of allocating resources. At the moment the basis for these decisions is questionable. Without effective evaluation of interventions the only parameter will be financial and this may not reflect in any way therapeutic effectiveness in terms of enhanced quality of life or service provision to clients. If the allocation of resources is to be considered in terms other than financial, therapists must establish appropriate methods of assessment and evaluation to use alongside economic measures.

Social factors

Social factors effect service provision and uptake at two levels, the allocation of resources and, at an individual level, the uptake of services. One of the major factors influencing accessibility to or uptake of services is social class. The inequalities in health care were highlighted for the first time by the publication in 1980 of the *Black Report* which showed how people in lower socioeconomic classes had less access to services.

Social factors also influence the resources allocated to specific services and this is especially apparent within the voluntary sector where individuals are contributing directly to what they perceive to be needy charities. Priorities for a Social Services Department in areas of inner cities may be different from the priorities faced by a Social Services Department in a rural area and thus effect the allocation of resources.

Political factors

Political factors can influence directly service provision via legislation. This is typified by such acts as The Chronically Sick and Disabled Persons Act 1970; Disabled Persons (Employment Act) 1974 and the Disabled Persons Act 1986. These acts influence in various ways the services provided to people with a disability and place statutory obligations upon local authorities to provide specific services. The Disabled Persons Act of 1986 went further and has given disabled people the right to appoint advocates to represent them and to appeal against decisions they may not agree with.

As described there are many factors which can influence the effectiveness of a team approach to management of a chronic disease, some of which are dependent upon the team members themselves, some upon the role of the client in the team and some upon factors which are not directly within the control of either clients or team members. However, communication of information at all levels is identified as a most important component of team work and essential if clients are to play any role other than that of a passive recipient. The emphasis of the following chapters is upon how therapists can utilize their skills to, in many instances, act as facilitators working with clients to help them identify their needs and play a role in meeting these needs. These skills are fundamental to the profession of occupational therapy and form the basis of the profession. The following section will look more closely at the role of the occupational therapist.

THE ROLE OF THE OCCUPATIONAL THERAPIST

When describing the work of occupational therapists the one phrase which most therapists use is 'It is an holistic approach'. The basis of this approach stems from the foundation of the profession at the beginning of this century upon the way in which illness affected the occupational nature of humans and of the therapeutic potential of activity to restore or re-organize daily activity. At this stage in the development of the profession disease categories or medical management were not seen as central to the work of therapists.

The developments in the scientific basis of medicine has been identified as causing a major shift in emphasis for the profession, which was perceived as having no theoretical basis. Occupational therapy became more aligned to the medical model of care which brought conflict between the analytical scientific model of the medical profession and the humanistic model of occupational therapy. These two models are seen as being opposed. Kielhofner aligns the medical model of care to a closed system which states 'that any system can be ultimately understood by reducing it to its least common denominators and specifying the cause effect relationships between them' as opposed to an open system approach which 'is a composition of structures organized into a coherent whole that interacts with an environment and that is capable of maintaining and changing itself.' (Kielhofner, 1985).

Closer alignment with a medical model of care brought the emphasis of the profession more towards diagnostic categories and disease pathology and represents for many therapists an area of continuing conflict, that of trying to explain occupational dysfunction in pathological terms. Kielhofner argues that this emphasis has taken the profession away from its original theoretical premis and that a balance is now needed to be achieved in the profession between analytical science and conceptual humanism (Kielhofner, 1982).

The incorporation of some of the analytical model will enable therapists to develop the skills and tools necessary to evaluate the validity of therapeutic interventions. Thus strengthening the theoretical framework of the profession.

The holistic approach of occupational therapy offers several dimensions to the treatment of a person with rheumatoid disease.

The skills of therapists aim to facilitate maximum independence by assessing the physical, psychological and social factors relevant to the way in which each client functions in order to plan appropriate interventions. The contribution of the therapist to the clinical team is one of assessing and monitoring the disease progress and the effectiveness of interventions in terms of a client's functional ability. This role frequently takes therapists away from the hospital setting and into the client's own home or work environment enabling a realistic picture of a client's abilities to be compiled away from the simulated environment of a hospital.

Therapists may be involved in treating clients in either an in-patient or out-patient setting or in the community, each with a slightly different emphasis to their work. Usually, on an in-patient basis, therapists are aiming to rehabilitate a client who has been through an acute period either due to increased disease activity, surgical or other forms of therapeutic intervention, or is experiencing decreased ability to cope due to psychosocial reasons. Out-patient treatment is primarily concerned with the treatment of conditions which do not warrant hospital admission or the inclusion in educational groups aimed at conveying information regarding specific methods of management.

Community based therapists are primarily referred clients who have a specific functional problem with a view to assessment and planned intervention. Some therapists are also involved in the development of self-help groups and support groups which are community as opposed to hospital based.

For occupational therapists the process of treatment planning is initiated with a period of assessment which aims to build up a picture of the clients' abilities, areas of limitation, their perceived needs and priorities and those of their family and to use this information, along with that gained by other team members to identify an appropriate treatment plan. As such a treatment plan is a specific plan of action with stated aims and identified objectives which provides a measure of how and if those aims have been achieved. The active involvement of the client is essential in establishing and implementing this plan. It is likely that in relation to a client with rheumatoid disease the plan will need reviewing and altering during the course of the disease.

The specific modalities used by therapists working in the field of rheumatology are primarily focused on the active involvement of the client and their ability to identify their needs, problem solve and adapt to the changes required to live with a chronic disease. The main premise of occupational therapy is that given the opportunity clients have the ability to make choices and play roles other than those of dependency and passivity. The first section of this book explores the way in which therapists can use their skills to provide these opportunities focusing on the use of self-management programmes, self-help groups and counselling to convey information, provide support and enable clients to explore their feeling about the impact of rheumatoid disease and the ways in which they cope with its effects.

The second section goes on to examine specific techniques which can be used to assist clients in maintaining functional ability, considering energy conservation, pacing, joint protection, the use of assistive equipment, housing adaptation, personal and sexual relationships, relaxation, splinting and community care.

The potential for occupational therapists within the field of rheumatology is great. It is an area of clinical practice where the skills of therapists can be used to full potential providing the opportunity to use clinical skills, psychotherapeutic skills and to embark upon areas of research. The opportunity is given to work within a team and contribute a dimension to the team which is based upon the holistic approach to therapy and the potential of the client, as opposed to a disease oriented approach.

FURTHER READING

G. Kielhofner (1985) *A Model of Human Occupation* Williams and Wilkins, Baltimore.

A. Mosey (1986) *Psychosocial Components of Occupational Therapy* Raven Press, London.

4

Assessment

The process of assessment is an information gathering process which is embarked upon jointly by therapist and client. It enables a picture to be created which identifies the client's present situation, but also includes aspects of their past and how they perceive their future. The chronic progressive nature of rheumatoid disease means that this picture is never complete but is a part of a series which helps to identify the client's perceived areas of need, their goals and expectations and provides an indication of their medical condition and the changes in each of these elements. These elements once identified indicate possible methods of management, help to evaluate the effectiveness of any intervention and monitor the progress of the client and the disease.

To enable this picture to evolve a range of assessments are needed, which can involve a varying number of people, of clinical, functional, psychological and social factors. When collated this information is the basis upon which interventions are planned. Inevitably there will be some areas of overlap in the assessment of team members but effective communication should eliminate as much of this as possible.

As the process of assessment forms the basis for developing a management programme it is essential that the client is an active participant in this process. The development of the role which it is hoped that the client will assume is established within this initial period of assessment and is influenced by the relationship established between the client and team members. The information gathered during this process should be explained to the client so that they do not feel themselves a passive recipient of treatment planned around them but central to the whole process.

Inclusion of the client and, if appropriate the family, at this stage will provide an indication that the client is seen as an active participant in their treatment. An information gathering process which does not include establishing the clients' priorities, understanding, plans and expectations is only placing a thin sketch upon a canvas and missing out the most important element, that which contains the colour, adds definition and brings meaning to the sketch.

Closer consideration will be given to some of the specific assessments used in relation to rheumatoid disease.

CLINICAL ASSESSMENTS

These assessments can include

1. pain and stiffness;
2. joint tenderness;
3. range of movement;
4. radiological assessment;
5. laboratory investigations.

Radiological and laboratory assessments have been considered in a previous chapter.

Pain and stiffness

The experience of pain and stiffness is subjective and therefore the assessment of each is based either upon the subjective report of the client or the subjective observations of the clinician. The pain measures most frequently used are, visual analogue scales, five point scales, or specific pain questionnaires. Visual analogue scales provide a linear representation of pain. A line 10 cm long is shown to the client with one end marked 'no pain' and the other 'unbearable pain' and the client is asked to mark a point on the line which is representative of the pain they are experiencing at present, or the worst pain they have experienced that week etc. The distance from the 'no pain' end is then measured in centimetres and a numerical value given. Five point scales range from 1 = mild pain to 5 = unbearable pain and clients are asked to choose the number which they feel is appropriate to the level of pain they are experiencing.

These methods all measure pain intensity. 'It is clear, however, that to describe pain solely in terms of intensity is like specifying the visual world only in terms of light flux without regard to pattern, colour texture, and the many other dimensions of visual experience' (Melzack and Ward, 1982). Therefore more in depth questionnaires

Joint tenderness/joint swelling

N.B.: Tenderness is elicited on all joints by firm pressure over the joint margin with the exception of the four * joints where it is elicited by passive movement of the joint.

	Joint tenderness			Joint swelling		
	Right	Left	0 = Patient has no tenderness 1 = Patient complains of pain 2 = Patient complains of pain and winces 3 = Patient complains of pain, winces and withdraws 9 = Non-respondable joint	Right	Left	0 = No joint swelling 1 = Mild joint swelling 2 = Moderate joint swelling 3 = Marked joint swelling 9 = Non-respondable joint
Cervical spine: *	☐					
Temporomandibular:	☐	☐		☐	☐	
Sternoclavicular:	☐	☐		☐	☐	
Acromioclavicular:	☐	☐		☐	☐	
Shoulder:	☐	☐		☐	☐	
Elbow:	☐	☐		☐	☐	
Wrist:	☐	☐		☐	☐	
Metacarpophalangeal:						
First (thumb):	☐	☐		☐	☐	
Second:	☐	☐		☐	☐	
Third:	☐	☐		☐	☐	
Fourth:	☐	☐		☐	☐	
Fifth:	☐	☐		☐	☐	
Proximal interphalangeal:						
Thumb:	☐	☐		☐	☐	
Index:	☐	☐		☐	☐	
Middle:	☐	☐		☐	☐	
Ring:	☐	☐		☐	☐	
Little:	☐	☐		☐	☐	
Hip: *	☐	☐				
Knee:	☐	☐		☐	☐	
Ankle:	☐	☐		☐	☐	
Talocalcaneal: *	☐	☐		☐	☐	
Midtarsal: *	☐	☐		☐	☐	
Metatarsophalangeal:						
First:	☐	☐		☐	☐	
Second:	☐	☐		☐	☐	
Third:	☐	☐		☐	☐	
Fourth:	☐	☐		☐	☐	
Fifth:	☐	☐		☐	☐	

Figure 4.1 The Ritchie Articular Index.

have been developed which aim to identify the quality of pain experienced by clients. The McGill pain questionnaire is an example of this which comprises lists of descriptors, words that describe the sensory, affective and evaluative aspects of pain, and present pain intensity rated from 0–5 (Melzack, 1975).

Joint tenderness

The Ritchie Articular Index was developed by Dorothy Ritchie, an occupational therapist, and colleagues, and is a scoring system to indicate joint tenderness (Figure 4.1) (Ritchie *et al.*, 1968). The assessment is carried out by the clinician palpating the joints and observing and scoring the client's response.

1. The patient feels no pain or tenderness.
2. The patient feels pain and says so.
3. The patient feels pain and winces.
4. The patient feels pain, winces and withdraws.

The collective scores are added together on completing the assessment providing a numerical indication of the amount of pain and tenderness a client is experiencing. This initial assessment acts as a baseline and can be used to monitor the effectiveness of any interventions being used. The assessment requires no equipment and is straight forward to perform. It is important that the same person carries out the assessment on each occasion as different assessors may use differing amounts of pressure when palpating a joint.

Musculoskeletal examination

It is not intended in this text to describe a full musculoskeletal examination as this is well documented in other texts, see recommended reading. The main composites of such an examination are, first to observe. Initially, observations can be made regarding a client's gait, posture, pallor, etc. Closer observations of specific joints may identify inflammation, the skin may be red, or odematous and deformities may be present. Palpating the joint will identify synovial proliferation, the presence of nodules and effusion and an indication of tenderness and pain.

Passive range of movement is tested by the therapist placing each joint through a full range of movement while the client is relaxed, as opposed to an active range of movement in which the client moves the joints through their range. There may be a difference in the range of movement achieved by each method. The stability of the joint may also be examined to detect signs of instability, subluxation or dislocation.

It is important that the time of day at which the assessment was taken is noted, as a client who has travelled to the department on public transport on a cold day in the morning for the first visit and is given a lift in the afternoon for the second visit may show an increase in range of movement which may not be due totally to therapist intervention. There is also a degree of inter-observer error with the use of instruments such as a goniometre, the exact positioning of the goniometre varying between therapists, so the same therapist should, wherever possible, complete the assessments.

Functional assessments

Functional assessments are a crucial component in the assessment of a client with rheumatoid disease reflecting the effect of impairment in terms of disability and handicap. This area of assessment is frequently undertaken by occupational therapists. The assessment is primarily an information gathering process and as such 'measures functional ability independent of other factors. Examination of the aetiology of dysfunction should be done independently of the measurement of function' (Liang and Jette, 1981). Therefore having completed an assessment an indication of a client's ability and disability is given but the process of assessment in isolation provides no causal explanation or statement of where to proceed to. As such a functional assessment can not be seen in isolation of assessment of client's needs, and goals or of clinical assessments.

The development of functional assessments has been identified as comprising three stages:

1. 1920–1940 to reimburse an impaired person for the loss of function;
2. 1940–1960 to provide more comprehensive and effective services to impaired people;
3. 1960–1983 to demonstrate accountability within all levels of the human service network (Halpern and Fuhrer, 1984).

These stages are not seen as developing in such a way that one stage replaces another but rather as a cumulative process. Assessment of function is a complex issue which remains in need of clarification, definition and standardization. Lack of clarity exists as to whether assessments are addressing issues related to impairment, disability or handicap and terminology is used frequently in an undefined way. There is a need to identify the composites of function and what is meant by a functional assessment. Until agreement is reached as to what constitutes activities of daily living it is not possible to construct a standard assessment. At the moment therapists use a wide range of assessments which comprise different activities. Methods of measurement also vary greatly as do processes for gathering the information. This leads to many questions relating to the reliability and validity of assessments.

Functional assessment is defined as 'the measurement of purposeful behaviour in interaction with the environment, which is interpreted according to the assessment's intended use' and from this definition seven key terms have been identified: measurement; purposeful; behaviour; environment; interaction; intended use and interpretation (Halpern and Fuhrer, 1984).

The way in which function is measured and the degree of the measurement detail is extremely variable. Methods of measurement include interview, observation, self-assessment and rating scales. The precision with which function is measured also varies. Five criteria have been identified as essential components of an assessment tool.

1. Allow quantification.
2. Have validity.
3. Have reliability.
4. Standardized data collection procedures.
5. Measurement precision (Liang, 1981).

Measurement scales are used to quantify or identify and comprise four scales; nominal; ordinal; interval or ratio (as reviewed by Eakin, 1989). A nominal scale is a descriptive category such as name, address, sex and race. The numbers given to the categories are merely labels and cannot be used as the basis for statistical calculations.

Steinbrocker and colleagues developed a classification of functional capacity in rheumatoid arthritis by identifying four classes (Steinbrocker, Traeger and Batterman, 1949). This is an example of an ordinal scale.

Class 1 Complete functional capacity with ability to carry on all usual duties without handicaps.

Class 2 Functional capacity adequate to conduct normal activities despite handicap of discomfort or limited mobility of one or more joints.

Class 3 Functional capacity adequate to perform only few or none of the duties of usual occupation or of self-care.

Class 4 Largely or wholly incapacitated with patient bedridden or confined to wheelchair, permitting little or no self-care.

Interval scales have the characteristics of ordinal scales but the distance between the categories can be measured in standard units. An interval scale does not have a fixed zero point and so numbers can only be added or subtracted. The ratio scale is the most sophisticated scale having a fixed zero point enabling all arithmetical procedures to be carried out. The problems around devising a rating scale of functional ability are immense and have been summarized by Eakin (1989).

Many functional scales are rated as the Stanford Index; 0 = able to complete task without difficulty; 1 = with difficulty; 2 = with some help from another person and 3 = unable to do (Fries *et al.*, 1980). The assumption is that each activity has the same value and so being unable to open a push button car door has the same value as being unable to get on and off the toilet, or being unable to use a pen or pencil the same value as being unable to walk outdoors on flat ground. Eakin states that many of these scales have been treated as fixed ratio scales and that it is erroneous to use these scales to calculate whether a client has improved as much as another client because:

1. the same score for different patients does not indicate that they are independent in the same activities;
2. two patients might improve equally, by, say, 5 points but one might move from dependent to partially dependent whilst the other might move from partially dependent to fully independent in five activities (Eakin, 1989).

It is also feasible that two clients can be scored as independent in feeding when one of them is independent as long as the meal is placed in front of them on the table and the other is independent not only in feeding but also in the preparation of the food. There remains a large amount of work to be completed in relation to the measurement of functional activities and the clarification, on an international level, of what constitutes activities of daily living.

The validity and reliability of the assessment has also to be established. Validity refers to measuring what the assessment purports to measure and this can be demonstrated by construct, content and criterion validity. In relation to activities of daily living it is difficult to demonstrate criterion validity as there is no accepted definition of what constitutes activities of daily living or a standard rating with which to compare. Content validity refers to the degree to which the assessment measures, in this case, activities of daily living and construct validity refers to the overall construct being investigated, i.e. activities of daily living; all the subsets must relate to this construct.

Reliability refers to the consistency of the results obtained, so if the same client completes the assessment twice, and the result is the same and if two assessors administer the same test to the same client do they achieve the same results? These refer to test re-test reliability and inter-observer reliability.

Reviews of literature indicate that this is an area in which much work is still needed, to define what is meant by activities of daily living thus providing the basis for a construct of a standard assessment, to validate assessments being used within the country of use, many assessments have been developed in the United States and modification may be required for use in this country, and to raise the standard of assessments carried out by therapists. The use of locally designed assessments and checklists does not provide valid and reliable assessments.

Occupational therapists must be carrying out, as a profession, a vast amount of functional assessments, it is disturbing to note the size of contribution they have made to this field of work. It is hoped that with the need to validate practice becoming recognized more widely this situation will change. The conclusion of a review of problems with assessments of activities of daily living leaves food for thought:

> The more occupational therapists who use the same assessments the easier it becomes to evaluate and compare treatment methods and outcomes. Without such measures, occupational therapists can never prove their true worth as members of the rehabilitation team   (Eakin, 1989).

This issue is perhaps appropriate for the special interests groups now emerging to consider and has indeed begun to be addressed by some of them.

Check lists are one of the most common forms of assessments used by therapists and comprise lists of activities against which the client's level of ability is noted. Thus the application of information gained via the use of a check list is limited to use with an individual by an individual.

The aim of the assessment should be identified before the process is embarked upon. Without answering the question 'why am I carrying out this assessment?' it is impossible to ensure that the appropriate assessment is being used, elements may be missing which are essential to fulfilling the aim or inappropriate methods of assessment may be used. There should be no such thing as a 'routine' assessment which is conducted without questioning the rationale and appropriateness of the process.

Behaviour is the object of the assessment and can be effected by impairment, disability and handicap. The International Classification of Impairment Disability and Handicap is as follows (World Health Organization, 1980).

- Impairment in the context of health experience is any loss or abnormality of psychological, physiological or anatomical structure or function.
- Disability is any restriction or lack (resulting from an impairment) of ability to perform an activity in the manner or within the range considered normal for the human being.
- Handicap is a disadvantage for an individual, resulting from an impairment or a disability, that limits or prevents the fulfilment of a role that is normal (depending on age, sex and social and cultural factors) for that individual.

Thus a chain of events can be identified starting with disease which leads to pathology and impairment. The term impairment refers to a biological process. When performance is affected by impairment the behavioural consequences become a disability and if this disability effects the performance of specific roles and places an individual at a disadvantage relative to others it leads to a handicap.

However, it must be remembered that each stage does not necessarily lead onto the next. Within the clinical field this fact is demonstrated frequently. On clinical examination a client may be present with greatly impaired anatomical structures of the hand. If a functional assessment is then carried out the functional ability of the client may be only affected slightly and there may be little or no evidence of disability or handicap. Clients with gross hand deformity have often demonstrated their ability to produce the most intricate and beautiful work. Impairment, disability and handicap can only be demonstrated in the context of the individual as they are subjective terms.

The effect of the environment in which the assessment is carried out may have a bearing on the results of the assessment and should always be borne in mind when the data is interpreted. However, several problems have been raised in relation to the measurement

59

and evaluation of function in different environments (Kelman and Willner, 1962). These mainly related to the variability and reliability of test performance and how these can be affected by the test environment, the motivation of the client and the interaction of the client and the evaluation setting. If a client's functional assessment in a hospital setting is different to an assessment at home which is used as the outcome criteria? A situation which has been observed in relation to clients with rheumatoid disease is a decline in function on returning home after a period of bed rest in hospital. It is difficult to say whether this is due to a difference in disease process, or the increased demands being placed upon a client at home. Therapists must ask themselves what information is really obtained about the way in which a client functions when assessed in a hospital environment and what relationship this bears to the client's overall functional ability. Can a single functional assessment reflect the impact of a disease which is so variable in nature and if not, how many assessments is it necessary to complete and in how many different environments to gain a realistic picture of functional ability?

Although an indication can be provided of the client's functional ability, thought should be given to the large number of variables which have been introduced into the assessment. The client is being asked to carry out activities in a simulated environment, many hospital bathrooms, for example, bear little relation to a bathroom in a client's home. The effect of being asked to conduct activities in front of a healthcare professional may introduce an element of not wanting to appear in need of help and tolerating more pain than if the client had been carrying out the activity alone or of not wanting to 'fail'.

A classic example of this is clients who claim mobility allowance and at the assessment make an effort to walk as far as they can in order to 'do their best' giving an unrealistic picture of their level of mobility. As a consequence their eligibility for the allowance can be questioned. It is easy for professionals to make valued judgements based on an assessment which bears little relation to the client's long-term level of functional ability and this factor should always be borne in mind, especially when making decisions on the appropriateness of assistive equipment or housing adaptations.

The other side of this coin is the dependent client who during assessment appears to be functioning at a higher level than is reported by other members of the family. The motivation to carry out activities is provided by the presence of the therapist and this motivation disappears on return home.

Studies have demonstrated a difference when assessments obtained from self-administered questionnaires were compared with an interview conducted by an occupational therapist. Patients were more willing to admit difficulties in a questionnaire than they were in a personal interview (Spiegel, *et al.*, 1985).

A continuation of this element of assessment is the interaction between a client's behaviour and the environment. Everyone's functional ability is influenced by the environment, different environments bring different demands, levels of motivation, stimulation and expectations. The functional demands for an elderly person living at home are far greater than those placed upon an elderly person living in residential care. Environments are often associated with specific roles and the behavioural components of those roles are adopted when entering into the environment, i.e. worker, parent, friend, patient. A difference in functional performance in elderly clients was observed when formally assessed in a hospital and in their residential home and when staff observed their functional ability as part of the daily routine. Different scores were obtained from the different assessments highlighting the variability in performance in different environments (Kelman and Willner, 1962).

The intended use of the data collected during assessment should be identified before the assessment is carried out alongside the purpose of the assessment. This can influence the amount of detail needing to be obtained from the assessment. The data may be used to plan an individual client's treatment programme, as the basis for planning service provision for a unit's strategic plan, or for the use of cost benefit analysis or as a component of a research project to evaluate the effectiveness of a specific intervention. Each of these situations demands different levels of information which must be established prior to the assessment taking place.

An assessment should specify the technique for administering the assessment and collecting and recording the data. An assessment which has been validated within a hospital population does not necessarily transfer to use with clients in a community setting and vice versa. Some of the most common forms of administering assessments include a guided interview, self-administered questionnaire, observation and performance testing. The precision of measurement refers to the degree of change which can be detected using the assessment. Some of the functional assessments used are not always sensitive enough to pick up changes in disease activity due to interventions such as the use of non-steroidal anti-inflammatory drugs.

61

One functional assessment which is used frequently by clinicians in clinical trials is the Disability Scale of the Health Assessment Questionnaire developed at the Stanford Arthritis Centre (Fries *et al.*, 1980). This has been shown to have validity and be reliable. But if the components of this assessment are examined there are few elements which a therapist might expect to change for a client having undergone knee replacement surgery. More significant changes may however be seen in relation to levels of pain and range of movement.

The final component of assessment is the way in which the data is interpreted in relation to its intended use. The interpretation of the data, in respect of treatment planning, may be influenced by other elements such as psychological and social factors relating to the client. Therapists, having established levels of function, will want to determine the reasons why areas may be affected and establish a programme aimed at increasing functional ability in relation to specific tasks. If the assessments are being used as a component of a research project the data may be subjected to a series of statistical analysis.

The lack of clarity, validity and reliability surrounding the assessment of function is, perhaps, an indication of the complexity of the nature of the assessment. The basis for gaining an element of understanding may be at an individual level compiling individual case studies. It is only when the framework of understanding on an individual level is obtained by consistently using valid and reliable assessments that data can be collated and interpreted across groups and perhaps contribute to a greater understanding of the impact of the underlying disease and pathology of a chronic progressive disease. While therapists continue to use locally designed checklists or assessment forms they contribute little to the understanding of the basis of their profession, and the effectiveness of their interventions.

Areas of function covered in assessment

Assessments of activities of daily living cover a broad spectrum of activities and usually include the following areas of function:

1. Transfers
   Chair;
   Bed;
   Toilet;
   Bath.

2. Personal care

  Dressing, managing fastenings, shoes, getting clothes from cupboards and drawers;
  Washing face;
  Washing body;
  Washing hair;
  Cleansing after using the toilet;
  Application of make-up;
  Shaving;
  Oral hygiene;
  Care of nails;
  Combing hair;
  Coping with menstrual cycle;
  Personal relationships.

3. Mobility

  Walking, inside and outside, on rough and smooth surfaces;
  Climbing steps and stairs;
  Access to house;
  Driving;
  Using public transport.

4. Home management

  Cooking
    making a drink;
    making a snack;
    preparing a meal;
  Housework
    washing;
    ironing;
    cleaning;
    managing plugs and sockets;
  Shopping;
  Using taps;
  Opening jars, bottles and tins.

5. Eating

  Use of cutlery;
  Taking cup to mouth.

6. Communication

  Writing;
  Using a telephone;
  Handling money.

7. Employment

  Mobility to and from work;

Mobility around the place of work;
Ability to carry out work.
8. Leisure activities
Ability to pursue hobbies.

This is not an exhaustive list and only serves to give an indication of areas of function which should be considered during assessment. The initial assessment serves to identify areas where problems exist. These specific areas are then investigated further to identify the cause of the problem and possible solutions. The assessment is also backed up with information from the initial interview which provides background information about the client and their family, their social situation etc.

HEALTH STATUS QUESTIONNAIRES

Health status questionnaires have been developed which take a multi-dimensional view of assessment, some have been specifically developed for use with clients with rheumatoid disease. One such scale is the Arthritis Impact Measurement Scale, AIMS (Meenan, *et al.*, 1982). This scale was designed to measure several dimensions of rheumatoid disease and contains nine scales, mobility, physical activity, dexterity, household activities, activities of daily living, anxiety depression, social activity and pain. The questionnaire is self-administered and has been shown to be reliable and valid in use with clients with rheumatoid arthritis, osteoarthritis, systemic lupus erythematosis and sero-negative variants. The Stanford Disability Questionnaire is another example of a multi-dimensional assessment and has five dimensions, death, discomfort, disability, drug of therapeutic toxicity and dollar cost, each of which has been broken down into components (Fries *et al.*, 1980). The functional component of the assessment has already been discussed.

PSYCHOLOGICAL ASSESSMENT

It is essential that therapists gain an appreciation of the psychological impact of rheumatoid disease upon the clients with whom they are working. This will be gained informally during the process of initial interview or assessments. If a client is exhibiting high levels of anxiety, stress or depression referral to a clinical psychologist may be indicated. This referral may result in the use of formal psychological assessments to identify in more detail the nature and extent of the client's problem and the most appropriate form of management.

An overall assessment of the client's psychological state can be obtained by asking pertinent questions and actively listening to the response. Asking the client how their life has changed since the onset of the disease will provide some information about the impact of the disease on the client's way of life and lead into a discussion of how these changes have been coped with both for the individual and their family.

It is also important to identify what factors are important in the client's life, what their hopes and expectations for the future are and how these equate with living with a chronic disease. This may identify whether the client is still going through a bereavement process and denying the long-term implications of the disease because 'it is going to go away', whether the responses are appropriate to the stage of disease which the client has reached and the effects of the disease to their lifestyle. Asking the client what they understand about arthritis will give an indication of their knowledge about the disease and how they think it will progress. The way in which clients cope with the pain they experience is also an important factor to establish and how this affects the way they function.

Asking appropriate questions and listening carefully to the response provides a good indication of the psychological problems a client may be experiencing, and an indication as to whether referral to a psychologist or far less frequently a psychiatrist is indicated. Depression, stress, anxiety and bereavement are normal responses to the onset and progression of a chronic disease which has chronic pain, leads to alteration in body image, functional ability and changes in lifestyle. It is when these symptoms in themselves begin to affect a client's functional ability and physical well being that problems arise. Interventions are directed frequently towards addressing problems once they arise, perhaps more thought should be given to the way in which interventions can be used to prevent these problems arising in the first place.

SOCIAL FACTORS

The impact of rheumatoid disease on the social network and relationships of a client will vary and depend upon the effect of the disease, both physically and psychologically on the client and the responses of others to these changes. Social contacts can reduce due to a vast number of reasons including limited mobility, pain and fatigue, loss of roles which include social contacts such as leaving work, decreased income, and withdrawal due to embarrassment at appearance.

A disproportionate amount of time may be given to purely functional aspects of living and leisure and social activities compromised as a result. This change can occur quite slowly and may not be apparent. In one group meeting clients were considering aspects of pacing and time management and assessing how such time had, that week, been spent on different activities and discussing things they used to do. One of the participants was horrified when she actually worked out what she was doing with her time and compared the mix of activities with that of a few years ago. She had never realized how many social activities she had stopped and in many instances could not think of the reasons why when she was still mobile and able to get out and about. The change had been so gradual that it had not been noticed.

Family dynamics can be altered fundamentally by the onset of a chronic disease in one family member, some of these factors have already been discussed. During assessment it is necessary to ascertain the amount of support a client receives from family and friends and whether this support is adequate or whether the use of community services are needed to assist with functional problems. The support given to a family caring for a dependent client can be a fundamental component in the length of time they are able to care for the client at home negating the need for admission to long-term care. Factors such as respite care should be discussed as well as other forms of relief to provide the carer with time to themselves.

The responsibility for the care of a family can also fall upon one parent as well as maintaining the family income. When a family is young and there are teenagers about the home support services frequently are not available as family members are expected to take on a share of the work. The reality can be very different and the pressure placed upon one partner can be immense. If appropriate this matter should also be discussed with the whole family to try and spread the work more evenly. Therapists should check whether a client is in receipt of benefit and if not whether this is appropriate and needing referral to a social worker.

THE PROCESS OF OCCUPATIONAL THERAPY ASSESSMENTS

Several stages lead up to carrying out an assessment, referral, initial interview and then assessment. The receipt of a referral leads on to an initial interview which identifies areas of need which are then assessed in a more specific way. The form that specific assessments take is varied and will include observation, activity analysis and the use of standardized tests.

The process of assessment enables a therapist to

1. identify the client's physical, psychological and social needs;
2. identify factors which may influence these needs;
3. gauge the client's understanding of their condition;
4. form a baseline for treatment;
5. identify short- and long-term goals;
6. plan appropriate treatment programmes and techniques;
7. evaluate the effectiveness of interventions;
8. modify treatment when appropriate;
9. monitor the course of the disease.

Referral

The source of the referral will include ward rounds; out-patient clinics; general practitioners; colleagues; community support services; family and self-referral. The information included in this may be broad, 'this lady is having problems coping' or specific requesting an assessment of hand function. The problem identified in the referral, especially if received from a client, may bear no relation to the main problem eventually identified by assessment as clients may feel they need some help but not be exactly sure what, or may feel unable to express their problem in an initial referral.

The information received may be supplemented with information from the medical notes, if available. While some therapists may feel ill-prepared if no further information is available they do have the advantage of approaching the assessment with no preconceived ideas about the client, which have been based upon the subjective comments of other colleagues.

67

Initial interview

The initial interview forms the basis of future relationships between client and therapist and enables a rapport to begin to develop. The therapist needs to obtain specific information during this interview which is therefore a guided conversation during which both client and therapist give and receive information. Therapists should be aware of the possible stress and anxiety clients may experience during this process. For a client this may be the first contact they have had with a healthcare professional and they may be unclear as to what this encounter may entail. Situations do occur where clients feel they are being tested, an example of this is a home visit prior to hospital discharge. These can be perceived as tests which are either passed or failed and upon which a decision will be taken regarding a client's ability to cope at home. This can place undue pressure on a client, especially if they have been in hospital for a long period of time, and may affect their functional ability.

The information that clients are being asked to give is often personal and frequently highlights areas of inability. Voicing limitations and talking about previous levels of function may emphasize areas of great personal loss which have never been vocalized before. The onus is therefore upon the therapist to create an environment in which information is communicated in a positive way.

The approach of the therapist is fundamental to future relationships with the client and forms the foundation upon which many of the occupational therapists' interventions are based. 'The skill of the therapist lies in the ability to guide a conversation without being too directive or dismissive and to show both empathy and the ability to listen actively'. Whilst it is impossible to avoid discussing areas of limitation, areas of skill and potential should also be discussed and reinforced. This is summarized as 'providing the right atmosphere, to be a good listener and to ask only the questions that help the client tell their own story' (Trombly, 1983).

Wherever possible the initial interview should be carried out in an environment which is free from distractions and comfortable. Therapists working in the community are able to carry out the whole process in the ideal environment for the client, their own home. The client has a greater feeling of security and, as the therapist is a guest, control. In the hospital environment the client is placed in an unfamiliar environment over which they have little control. Few wards offer privacy and many interviews are carried out by the patients bed. Although drawing the curtains offers visual privacy many therapists will have experienced silence descending in a ward when a particularly personal subject is being discussed.

During the first few days of hospital admission a person will have undergone several physical examinations, a series of clinical investigations and have answered many repetitive questions. Therapists should remember this fact and not attempt a long assessment following on from another member of the team, if at all possible.

Assessment

The timing and content of an assessment will vary on the needs which have been identified in a referral or following an initial interview. When interpreting the outcome of an assessment, however, therapists should consider carefully the information gathered. The variability of disease activity is reflected in a client's functional ability and therefore assessments must be considered in the light of this. A functional assessment carried out in the morning may vary considerably from one carried out in the middle of the afternoon. The information gathered from an assessment at home may vary from that gathered in a hospital setting. If a series of assessments are being carried out as a means of identifying progress following treatment interventions it is essential that these assessments are carried out at the same time of day and if possible by the same therapist.

If a client has been in hospital for an extended period of time, undergone operative procedures or for any other reason their ability to cope at home is in question a pre-discharge assessment may be carried out. Pre-discharge assessments are carried out to:

1. ensure the client has achieved a level of function to maintain themselves at home;
2. determine the amount of support needed upon discharge and identify the appropriate agencies;
3. identify the need for the provision of assistive equipment or adaptation and determine the most appropriate type given environmental limitations;
4. enable community agencies to meet the client and their family prior to discharge and establish communication with hospital staff.

Therapists carrying out home assessments should always be aware of the pressures upon the client when undertaking such a visit. The thought of returning home for an hour's visit, especially after a long absence, can be extremely frustrating and upsetting. Pressure can be added by a feeling of having to pass a test before being allowed home and fear of failure. The amount of activities to be completed in this time is also unrealistic and demanding and this should be recognized by the therapist. An imminent discharge can bring a range of feeling for the client, especially if they live alone, ranging from happiness and fear to anxiety and loneliness.

Therapists should also consider the implications of the information obtained during such a visit. The information will help to identify specific equipment which may be considered within the environment in which it will be used and to provide an indication of a client's functional ability in relation to one or two activities. Home assessments can also provide an opportunity for community support staff who will be involved in the patient's treatment when discharged to meet the client and gain some understanding of the problems the client may be experiencing. Therapists will be all too familiar with the home assessment where there are so many staff involved that completing any meaningful assessment of functional ability becomes impossible. There is a lot to be said for keeping staff to a minimum and communication being improved by community staff having a greater involvement in pre-discharge hospital based work.

However, the long-term reality of coping at home cannot be simulated in such a visit and for this reason post-discharge visits may be appropriate to ascertain the long-term problems clients may be experiencing. Admission to hospital, for many clients, represents a significant reduction in activity. Some clients have expressed disappointment and frustration regarding their level of function and increase in pain when they have been at home for a few days. Their level of function has returned to that prior to admission. The feeling of well-being when laying in a hospital bed can be false and unrealistic and lead to disappointment and fear a few days after returning home, for the client and their family. This can be a time when support is felt to be lacking after the security of a hospital ward where someone, whether staff or another patient, was usually around to talk with.

The process of assessment is fundamental to the planning of a treatment programme. It is an information gathering exercise aimed at building up a picture of the client's physical, psychological and social needs and then, with the client, placing them in an order of priority to work towards addressing. In the long-term it will enable information to be gathered providing a picture of the progression of the disease and its impact upon the individual. The format of assessments is varied, some components of the assessments being standardized, valid and reliable and others being highly subjective. The challenge for therapists remains to identify and use standard and reliable assessments enabling the information collated to be used to evaluate the effectiveness of interventions. Without the use and availability of valid and reliable assessment procedures the evaluation of interventions becomes meaningless. The completion of the assessment procedures enables areas of need to be identified and subsequent chapters will discuss interventions used by occupational therapists to address some of the issues.

FURTHER READING

C. Partridge, R. Barnitt (1986) *Research Guidelines, A Handbook for Therapists*, Heineman Physiotherapy, London.
O. Payton (1988) *Research: The Validation of Clinical Practice*, 2nd edn, F.A. Davis Company.
C. Trombly (1983) *Occupational Therapy for Physical Dysfunction*, Williams and Wilkins, Baltimore.

5

Developing skills

As a therapist working in the field of rheumatology one of the most fundamental aspects of the work is the ability to assist people in developing some of the skills necessary to cope with the challenge of a chronic disease. In some situations this may entail the development of existing skills and abilities while in others new skills may need to be acquired. The holistic approach of occupational therapy enables a wide range of skills to be explored with clients ranging from concepts of pacing and joint protection to aspects of coping with stress and anxiety. This may entail working either on an individual or group basis. The skills of occupational therapists extend far beyond addressing the purely physical components of a disease and the potential to use these skills is at its greatest in assisting clients to meet some of the challenges posed by chronic disease.

The variability and unpredictability of rheumatoid disease makes acquiring a set of coping strategies difficult. A condition which is static, while initially posing many difficulties, enables specific skills to be developed to address needs. The response of a client with rheumatoid disease has to remain flexible as the condition is moving between periods of acute and chronic disease, each bringing different problems and needs. The progressive nature of the disease also requires some reappraisal in the type of response used as differing levels of pain and functional ability pose new problems.

The amount of time clients spend in contact with healthcare professionals is fractional in terms of the overall duration of the disease. Therefore clients need to know how to utilize the resources available to them to try to address problems as and when they occur. To do this the transference of information and the development of skills are essential. The resources available to clients and the ways in which these resources are utilized will vary considerably. The main focus for planning a management programme is the identification of the client's perceived needs, the resources available to the client and the most appropriate way, for that client, in which these resources can be used. A client with a large social network may seek support from within this network whereas a client living alone may join a self-help group to find the same level of support.

The aim of this section is to give consideration to some of the settings in which information can be communicated and coping skills developed. The potential use of self-management programmes, self-help groups and counselling will be discussed.

PROVISION OF INFORMATION

The provision of information within the field of healthcare is developing as recognition of the need to include clients in the promotion of health and the management of chronic disease is growing. The main emphasis of many programmes is in the field of primary healthcare and preventative medicine aiming to provide the relevant information to enable people to make informed decisions regarding health matters. These programmes range from vaccination programmes to the promotion of healthy eating habits and anti-smoking campaigns.

The responsibility for health education is shared by government, statutory agencies, the voluntary sector, the media and each individual. Government responsibility is seen mainly in relation to the implementation of legislation and social reform. Statutory agencies and local authorities are responsible for the implementation and monitoring of government policy and for advising on strategies.

The voluntary sector is now playing a major role in the provision of information which is predominantly directed towards specific diseases and methods of coping with them. The large growth in information from the voluntary sector is, perhaps, an indication of the divergent beliefs between the voluntary sector, which is largely client led, and the statutory sector, which is largely professional led, regarding the need for information and the allocation of resources to meet this need.

The media, arguably, play the most important role in influencing public opinion on, and behaviour towards, health related topics, whether via advertising, reporting or dramatic representation of issues.

The individual is ultimately responsible for assimilating the information and deciding whether to follow or ignore recommendations. The adoption of a specific piece of information, while predominantly affecting the individual, can also influence the attitudes and behaviours of immediate and extended family and in some situations the wider community.

Information related to rheumatoid disease is provided on both a national level, via the Arthritis and Rheumatism Council and Arthritis Care, and on a local basis via self-help groups, voluntary organizations and healthcare professionals. This information is aimed at a varied audience which includes, clients with the disease, providing specific information, the general public, to increase understanding of the disease or raise money to fund research, and also at colleagues to increase their understanding of the needs of clients with rheumatoid disease.

As a therapist the expressed wish for information relating to health issues is frequently encountered. The development of self-management programmes is one way of meeting this need by conveying information in a structured way.

EDUCATIONAL PROGRAMMES

Before discussing the development and implementation of educational programmes it is necessary to consider the rationale behind the programmes and their aims. Programmes have been developed in many different forms and contain a wide variety of information. Some of the programmes have been specific and concentrate on providing information on one topic such as exercise programmes or precautions following joint replacement surgery and some are broad and cover a range of information on different topics.

One of the main criticisms of educational programmes is the discrepancy between aiming to provide choice and increase involvement and yet measuring their effectiveness in terms of compliance. This ambiguity is typified by the frequent occurrence in the literature of statements such as 'We recommend patient education as an effective means of helping patients to understand and hence comply with physicians' instructions as well as helping patients assume a greater responsibility for their own care.' (Kaye and Hammond, 1978). It is difficult to perceive how compliance and assuming more responsibility can be achieved within the same programme.

Programmes aimed at increasing compliance are developed along totally different lines and using different approaches to those aimed at increasing control and participation in decision making. The range of approaches can be described along a continuum which, at one end, starts with an overt aim to change behaviour and, at the other end, finishes with self-help. The role of healthcare professionals becomes less directive further along the continuum and the aim of increasing compliance remains very much towards the behaviour change end of the line. It is therefore essential that the aim of providing information is clearly identified so that the most appropriate approach can be identified along with the most appropriate information provided.

Given a range of information clients will adopt the information and use the resources which they feel are appropriate to themselves and their situation, exercising a degree of choice and control. Not enough work has been carried out to identify what clients perceive to be important or useful information and which coping strategies are more commonly adopted than others. The main bulk of studies have concentrated on the effectiveness of different formats of providing information, ways of increasing compliance and only in the last few years, the affect on psychosocial parameters.

The long-term implications of participating in educational programmes are yet to be identified. While behaviour change has been noted the duration of this change and the affects on the disease progress and levels of pain and functional ability remain a matter for debate. The evaluation of interventions is of paramount importance in an area where little is known about the effectiveness of treatment. It is essential therefore when planning a programme that effective methods of evaluation are identified.

It is also necessary to recognize that many factors influence behaviour and the provision of information about coping strategies and treatment regimes does not necessarily equate with the adoption or use of the information. The perceived appropriateness of the information, social and economic factors all influence whether a client will utilize it or not.

CHOOSING APPROPRIATE APPROACHES

A variety of approaches have been identified to utilize in educational programmes, a medical approach, behaviour change approach, educational approach, client directed approach and social change approach (Ewles and Simnett, 1985). The three approaches most frequently used by therapists are: the behavioural change, educational and client directed approach.

The behaviour change approach

The main emphasis of this approach is placed upon changing a person's behaviour and attitudes, i.e. adopting an exercise programme or weight reducing diet. The therapist is placed in the position of expert and provides instructions to be carried out explaining the rationale behind them. This places the therapist in a position of being directive and in control.

One of the criticisms of this approach is the concept of 'victim blaming' (Naidoo, 1986). This refers to the situation which arises if a client chooses not to adopt the recommended regime. If their condition deteriorates and they need to seek further assistance they may feel that they are to blame for the deterioration and expect to be greeted with the all telling 'I told you so' look. This can be a cause of not seeking help for fear of rejection or reprimand.

Therapists using this approach should be aware of this concept and question their own responses to clients who are deemed to be non-compliant. Many factors can cause people to not adopt new approaches not least the therapist's failure to set realistic aims which are specific to the client's needs and social situation, having expectations which are too high or priorities which are different from those of the client's.

Therapists should try to gain an understanding of factors which may influence client's behaviour and acknowledge their existence. Some of the socioeconomic factors affecting healthcare in Great Britain were highlighted in *The Black Report* (1980) which was compiled by the Working Group on Inequalities in Health set up in 1977 under the chairmanship of Sir Douglas Black. An assessment of this has been made by Townsend and Davidson (1985). It is factors such as these which are easy to overlook in a clinical setting and yet are fundamental to healthcare. Therapists may feel unable to agree with some of the reasons given by clients for not following treatment programmes but recognition and acknowledgement does not necessarily mean endorsement but may enable both therapist and client to respect each other's opinion and maintain channels of communication, leaving the door open should the client change their mind.

The client directed approach

This approach is the least directive approach for professionals involved. Their role is seen as facilitatory and they give no sense of direction to the group. This approach may be used in counselling groups or in some forms of self-help groups. The use of this approach is seen infrequently in a medical setting and to some clients may pose a threat. The expectation of many clients regarding healthcare professionals is that they are perceived as being prescriptive, directive and in control. When confronted by someone who is perceived as providing no assistance and expecting you as a client to make decisions and a major contribution to the group clients can express anger, resentment and anxiety. Therapists skilled in group facilitation will be able to use their skills to work with the group to overcome these problems. The use of this approach needs much more time as the development of group cohesiveness, identification of needs and aims of the group will take longer to establish than with a more directive approach that has identified aims as a prerequisite to establishing the programme.

The educational approach

This approach is less directive than the behaviour change approach and more directive than the client directed approach placing more onus on the need to present information in as unbiased a way as possible. It aims for the client to gain an understanding of the issues discussed and emphasizes the client's ability to make decisions based upon the information gained.

As is common with concepts occupying the middle ground an area of grey exists where the other approaches meet and this approach can be used as a compromise. The behaviour change approach is blatant in its statement of intent to change behaviour and attitudes, the client directed approach is directly opposed to this and aims towards facilitating self-determination. The educational approach is a way of giving an element of choice while still maintaining some control over the group structure, content and process.

The main issue surrounding the use of this approach is the extent to which a degree of choice is allowed and what is meant by choice in this context. When a programme of information is evolved how much choice do therapists really aim to give clients? Is the information presented in an unbiased way?

Perhaps this compromise offers a range of options to both therapists and clients, offering therapists the opportunity to maintain some control and be seen in the light of 'professional' and yet still feeling that clients are having a significant say in the structure and content of the programme. It may also offer clients the opportunity to feel some degree of control and active participation while feeling that the therapists are still providing support and professional advice decreasing feelings of stress and anxiety about being asked to assume too much responsibility. The effectiveness of different approaches in relation to chronic disease has not as yet been established and is an area in which evaluation is needed urgently.

When developing an educational programme therapists need to consider the underlying rational behind the programme in order to choose the most appropriate approach. The approach chosen must reflect the thinking of all participants in the programme. If some team members feel unhappy using a client directed approach, needing to be directive, or do not have the skills necessary to facilitate group processes, group participants could end up confused about the role which they are being asked to adopt. They may be receiving contradictory information from group leaders.

USE OF EDUCATIONAL APPROACHES

The use of educational approaches in the management programmes of clients is encountered frequently. The aims, structure, content and approaches used in programmes are varied. Sometimes they are used on a one to one basis, sometimes on a group basis. Individualized programmes may be used when the information being conveyed is of relevance only to one person, such as a specific treatment regime. Group programmes are used frequently by therapists where a group of clients with broadly the same needs can be identified. In terms of information retention it has been suggested that individualized programmes produce a greater learning gain than group programmes (Lorish, Parker and Brown, 1985).

There are, however, other factors which may influence the choice of group work as opposed to individual programmes. The support that group members can gain from each other and from sharing experiences should not be underestimated. Most clients cope alone with the problems they encounter daily and can feel isolated in doing so. They may also feel that the problems they are encountering are unique to them as they have no gauge by which to measure them. While families are usually sympathetic and supportive there comes a time when clients feel unable to burden their families with the problems they have heard numerous times before. Bringing people with similar problems together in a group does provide an opportunity for the sharing of information and the discussion of problems with people who have a greater degree of empathy.

One dilemma which confronts therapists when formulating a programme based upon group work is whether or not group members should be at roughly the same stage in the disease process. Is it distressing for newly diagnosed clients to be involved in groups with clients who may have had the disease for several years, have developed deformities and have lost some aspects of function?

Three considerations have been identified in relation to group work carried out with people with multiple sclerosis (Pavlon, Harting and Davis, 1978). Contagious fears arose among group members whereby the clients who were less disabled by their condition were afraid of being made worse by being in contact with people whose condition was more advanced. This was seen as a 'natural extension and modification of a phenomenon seen in new groups universally' and such feelings were identified even in groups which were homogenous with regard to disease level. If the group members are self-selected then those members who do not wish to confront issues relating to their future will cease to attend and therapists can thus identify them and follow them up to ensure that they have not suffered any harm and offer alternative ways of receiving information if they so wish.

The positive effects of heterogeneous groups were identified as less disabled members 'spending less energy avoiding fearful thoughts of the future and less time avoiding situations in which they might be frightened in this way'. The groups which were comprised solely of less disabled members showed higher levels of anxiety as there was 'no discrete focus for their fears of deterioration'.

The inclusion of relatives is another issue which arises when planning programmes. There are advantages and disadvantages which need to be considered. The inclusion of relatives can be inhibitive for both clients and family members with regard to the expression of issues which may relate to family relationships. It is sometimes difficult to discuss problems which may be occurring within a relationship, or perceived lack of understanding if both partners are present. However, family members also have the need to be provided with information regarding the disease, its management and specific treatment regimes. Family support has been associated with client's adoption of specific regimes such as wearing splints, taking medication and exercising (Ferguson and Boyle, 1978; Oakes et al., 1970).

Three broad areas of educational work in rheumatology can be identified as:

1. clients having undergone the same operative procedure;
2. information relating to a specific treatment technique;
3. broad based self-management programmes.

Therapists have developed educational groups for clients who have undergone the same course of treatment, as in the case of joint replacement surgery. An example of this is a group which is developed for clients who have undergone hip replacement surgery. As the number of clients having hip replacement surgery increases therapists time is being taken up explaining to each person the precautions which it is necessary to take post-operatively and ways in which they can remain independent within these limitations. A more effective use of time is to develop a group programme of information, supplemented with a booklet to overcome the time-consuming repetition of information on an individual basis.

Groups may also be used to convey information regarding a specific treatment technique such as relaxation. This sort of programme would usually comprise more than one session to ensure that time is given for reinforcement and practice of the technique being taught.

The development of a self-management programme can meet the wider information needs of clients and usually contains information relating to a variety of issues. Such programmes are usually implemented by more than one member of the team, if not via direct involvement in groups then via input into the planning stage.

The planning of such work, whether on an individual or group basis and whether for one session or a programme of several sessions is essential and comprises several stages.

1. Identifying the client group.
2. Establishing their needs and expectations.
3. Developing aims and objectives.
4. Organizing content and identifying resources.
5. Planning methods of evaluation.
6. Implementing the programme.
7. Evaluation and if appropriate, revising the programme.

These various stages will now be discussed using the development of a self-management programme as an example.

Identifying client group

Referrals from consultants and discussion with clients attending a rheumatology out-patient clinic identified a need for information to be provided regarding different aspects of managing rheumatoid disease. This need was also voiced by clients who were admitted to the ward. Discussion with in-patients revealed a frustration that they were receiving information once admitted to the ward which they had not had access to as an out-patient and how much they would have valued this opportunity prior to admission. In-patients also related feelings of isolation and fear regarding coping with the disease and not knowing what help was available or what they could be doing to help themselves.

On this basis a self-management programme for clients attending out-patient clinic was developed to enable participants to have access to a variety of information related to coping with rheumatoid disease. This client group was identified as an expressed need from clients and a perceived need by therapists. It was decided that anyone attending out-patient clinic with rheumatoid disease could participate in the programme and participants were given the opportunity to bring along a family member.

Establishing needs and expectations

Having identified the client group it was necessary then to establish the needs of the group in a more precise fashion. It is essential that clients are approached in the development of a programme and their needs not assumed by the programme organizer. The needs identified by healthcare professionals do not always reflect the needs identified by clients and different priorities are placed upon different issues. A survey designed to compare the views of clients and professionals regarding the importance of different aspects of self-care showed that clients rated more highly aspects related to such things as exercise and energy conservation and that professionals rated the provision of assistive equipment, sexual counselling and drug treatment more highly than clients (Potts, Weinberger and Brandt, 1984). Therefore it should not be assumed that effective programmes can be planned without consultation with representatives from the group at whom the programme is aimed. Neither should it be assumed that because a person has had rheumatoid disease for ten years or been admitted to hospital that they have been in receipt of an abundance of information, this in many instances is not the case.

Clients' needs can be identified in various ways. Initially conversations with representatives of the specific group should provide information upon which a programme can be developed. It is worth considering, however, that the needs expressed by clients to therapists may not reflect totally what they feel. Clients may feel a need to say what they think the therapist would like to hear, or if this discussion is carried out on a group basis may reflect the needs of the most vocal and dominant group member. If a therapist feels that either factor is the case she may wish to follow up initial discussion with a questionnaire based upon these discussions. If the questionnaire is anonymous it may be a more accurate reflection of client need. It can also be circulated on a wider basis and therefore gain a more representative picture of the client group's wishes.

Simple questionnaires can provide a wealth of information to assist in programme development. They can provide an indication of programme content, venue, frequency, timing and inclusion of family members.

Alongside establishing the needs of client's it is also necessary to establish the needs of colleagues who are working with the client group. Their views regarding approaches, content and evaluation are essential and will also provide perceptions from a different view point. If the programme is being developed along a multi-disciplinary team approach other team members involved in the implementation of the programme should be involved in the planning.

While establishing needs it is necessary to establish the expectations of both colleagues and clients towards participation in the programme. The expectations of clients involved in a self-management programme can range from the information received making no difference at all, to being able to do more for themselves, to seeing a change in the underlying disease process. High expectations can be a cause of disappointment and evoke a sense of failure when expectations are not met. Therapists should be aware of the participants' expectations of the programme as this can assist in ensuring that the aims and objectives are explained initially, hopefully placing into context the expectations of the group organizers and the participants.

Developing aims and objectives

Once the background work has been completed it should be possible to establish the aims and objectives of the programme. In the development of a self-management programme there may be several levels of aims and objectives.

The overall aim of a programme may be to

develop a self-management programme for clients attending out-patient clinic which identifies a range of possible coping strategies and resources which may be of assistance in coping with rheumatoid disease, the programme being backed up with written information.

The objective being to

identify any effect participation in the programme had on disease parameters using a multidimensional assessment comprising valid and reliable measures.

While these were the overall aims and objectives for the programme being discussed more specific aims and objectives were developed for each session included in the programme. These should identify in a more precise way the aim of each session and the ways in which it is possible to identify whether or not these aims have been achieved. The overall aim of the programme will also identify the most appropriate approach to use. The above aim led to the development of a programme using an educational approach. A set programme was established based on identified needs of a representative group, but the programme was developed to provide scope for discussion and was flexible, to some extent, in content to meet the needs of different groups. However, it was not a client directed approach as time was not spent on working with each group to identify their needs and enable them to arrive at the direction they wished to take. The resources, especially therapist's time, were not available to use this approach and the programme would have been only available to a much smaller number of people.

Organizing content and identifying resources

Having established aims and objectives the content of the programme is identified more easily. The content will, to some extent, be dependent upon the resources available in terms of time, venue, finance, teaching materials and support. While considering group leaders it is worth considering the possibility of co-running groups with a person with rheumatoid disease. In an evaluation of self-management courses no difference was identified in outcome between groups which were therapist led and groups which had been led by lay people who had participated in a training course (Cohen and Lazarus, 1979).

If it is decided to develop teaching resources to compliment group sessions adequate time should be allowed in the preparation of the programme for this to be carried out. The production of teaching material, if done well, is a lengthy process.

Planning methods of evaluation

It is essential that some form of evaluation is carried out, as a minimum, to identify whether or not the stated aims and objectives are being achieved. The ways in which this is performed range from the use of questionnaires designed by the therapist to the use of valid and reliable measures. The use of pre-testing may identify more clearly any changes which may have taken place as a result of the intervention. A wealth of information can be made available to therapists if systematic evaluation of programmes is carried out preferably with valid and reliable measures. Information will be provided to enable the effectiveness of interventions to be identified, directions in which to progress work clarified and a degree of understanding of the management of the disease contributed to the body of knowledge being assimilated.

Implementing the programme

The following programme is an example of a programme used with out-patients with rheumatoid disease. The sessions were held on a weekly basis, each session lasting an hour and a half with a break for coffee and a change of position. Sessions 1, 3, 4 and 5 were led by an occupational therapist, session 2 by a physiotherapist.

Session 1   the disease process and its management

Aim   To enable participants to gain an understanding of the way in which rheumatoid disease affects their body and ways in which it is managed clinically.

Content
1. The structure of a synovial joint.
2. The way in which inflammation can effect this structure.
3. Systemic features of rheumatoid disease.
4. Medical management of the disease.
5. Other forms of management, including diet and homeopathy.

Session 2   the use of exercise

Aim   To enable participants to gain an understanding of the use of exercise programmes, how to adjust them according to disease activity and how to use heat and ice at home.

Content
1. The rationale behind the use of exercise.
2. The difference between range of movement, isometric and passive exercises.
3. Demonstration of and participation in a range of movement programme.
4. Explanation of how and when to use heat and ice.
5. Discussion on swimming and exercises to carry out in water.

Session 3   maintaining function

Aim   To provide information on maintaining function by pacing and the use of assistive equipment.

Content
1. Explanation of the concept of pacing.
2. Discussion on what is meant by rest, activity and exercise and how the three can be balanced.
3. Demonstration of some small items of assistive equipment.
4. Discussion on the use of equipment and its provision.

Session 4 *coping with rheumatoid disease*

Aim To provide the opportunity for participants to discuss how they cope with problems arising from rheumatoid disease and to identify possible resources which may be of assistance.

Content
1. Introduction from therapist about coping with pain and loss of function.
2. Open discussion from group members.

Session 5 *relaxation*

Aim To provide the opportunity for participants to discuss how they cope with stress and tension and participate in a period of relaxation.

Content
1. Continuation of previous week's discussion.
2. Discussion on how pain can cause tension.
3. Explanation of what relaxation entails and different methods relaxation session.

While this programme provides a brief outline it can give an indication of the type of programme which can be used. The onus of this programme was essentially on introducing and discussing basic concepts and ideas and providing participants with an insight into the potential they have to help themselves. The sessions were backed up with a booklet which had been produced in conjunction with the local Health Education Authority and compiled by various members of the team. The booklet comprised:

1. the disease process and management;
2. the use of exercise, with a fully illustrated exercise programme;
3. the use of heat and ice;
4. swimming;
5. pacing and energy conservation;
6. the use of assistive equipment;
7. coping with stress;
8. personal relationships;
9. employment;
10. mobility;

11. footwear and footcare;
12. local resources.

Each section gave basic information and practical advice. The section on local resources provided addresses of social service offices, local self-help groups etc. This programme was a basic introduction for group members and provided an opportunity for out-patients to meet with other people experiencing similar problems and to discuss some of their problems with other group members and therapists. It is worth relaying the fact that group members, via evaluation, felt that a person with rheumatoid disease should co-run the groups as they would have a greater understanding of problems and would also help to overcome some of the fear group members felt about coping with the future, i.e. they could talk to someone who has coped for a period of years. Some of the group participants still keep in touch with each other socially showing that the effects in terms of support can be long lasting.

Evaluation

Having implemented the programme the evaluation should be carried out, gathering the data together and its implications considered. The information gathered during evaluation may well identify areas of the programme which need revising or developing.

When considering the development of an educational programme it is also necessary to consider which medium is the most effective way of conveying the information, this will now be discussed.

THE USE OF DIFFERENT MEDIUMS

The range of mediums available to therapists to convey information has never been greater. The facility to communicate via the written or spoken word, slides or videos, or the use of computer programmes is now readily accessible to most therapists. Teaching materials are available on a national basis via various publishers as are audio visual materials. Local resources are usually available if therapists wish to develop their own specific packages. Mediums available include: pamphlets and booklets, workbooks, tapeslide programmes, cassette tapes and computer programmes. The potential of these different mediums has not, as yet been realized in relation to developing materials for clients to use, not only in departments but also in their own homes. Many of these mediums, with the exception of tapeslide programmes, are now accessible to a growing number of clients in their own homes. This means that learning can take place at the pace of the individual, it can be reviewed when necessary and is also available to other members of the family.

While therapist-led sessions convey information, the use of supplementary information means that clients can have access to information when they want it. Sometimes information conveyed may not be relevant immediately but several years later can be retrieved as necessary.

Pamphlets and booklets

A wide range of booklets are available on a national basis via the Arthritis and Rheumatism Council. Titles applicable to clients with rheumatoid disease include: *Rheumatoid arthritis explained*, *A new hip joint*, *Alternative medicine*, *Are you sitting comfortably?*, *Arthritis: sexual aspects and parenthood*, *Choosing shoes*, *Driving and your arthritis* and *Your home and your rheumatism*. These booklets provide information in a clear and concise format (Arthritis and Rheumatism Council). Therapists also produce frequently their own supplementary information to programmes they are developing. The standard of this literature varies from A4 sheets of typed information to illustrated and printed booklets. Before re-inventing the wheel it is worth establishing exactly what is available as the development of such materials is time consuming and costly.

Workbooks

Workbooks are encountered more frequently in the United States where the production of educational material tends to be more formalized with educationalists employed specifically to co-ordinate and develop educational activities within units. The information ranges from fact sheets about routine investigative procedures such as X-rays to management programmes for specific conditions. An example of this is *Rehabilitation Through Learning: Energy Conservation and Joint Protection. A Workbook for People with Rheumatoid Arthritis* (Furst, Gerber and Smith, 1982). This book comprises four sections: body positioning, rest, activity analysis and joint protection.

Each section outlines teaching objectives and provides information and practical suggestions. The information is followed by a series of worksheets for clients to complete and an evaluation checklist. Such books can be used in conjunction with therapist led sessions providing useful information as to how the client is using the information and how they are applying it to their daily routine. The practical application can act as a reinforcement of the written information.

Books

A growing number of publications are on general release which provide a variety of information regarding rheumatoid disease. Some have been written by therapists and clinicians and others by people with the disease or people involved in other forms of intervention, such as homeopaths or dieticians. As these publications are available through many libraries and local bookshops it is well worth therapists reviewing the publications so that the information presented is known about should clients refer to books which they have read. It may be appropriate for copies to be kept in the department.

Tapeslide programmes

Commercially produced programmes are now available on such topics as joint protection, medication and exercise programmes. While some therapists have embarked upon developing their own programmes the time involved may be prohibitive. The main draw back of this medium is that it is not as accessible as other mediums as the appropriate audiovisual equipment must be available, therefore its use is usually limited to wards and clinics. An advantage of this medium however is that it is accessible to clients who have reading difficulties, which the options mentioned previously are not.

Tapes

Probably one of the most widely recognized uses of tapes is in the teaching of relaxation techniques. They are relatively easy to prepare needing only a tape recorder and are easily reproducible. They are also a medium which a large proportion of clients will be able to use within their own homes. Tapes are also a useful way of supplementing information for people who have a visual impairment and who otherwise may not have access to written information.

Videos

The potential of videos is yet to be realized in relation to conveying information to clients. The cost of production and the availability of equipment may prohibit the development of videos within many departments. Again this is a medium which can be used within a growing number of clients' homes and is also a medium to which people can easily relate.

Computer programmes

The development of computer programmes as an educational medium is a new area for many therapists. As more departments are installing computers for use as a treatment medium or for departmental administration it is becoming a more widely available medium. As a medium it may deter some clients who feel unable to cope with new technology but for a certain group of clients it may prove ideal. It is an active learning process as responses to questions are required bringing a degree of involvement and challenge which other more passive mediums such as watching a slide programme lack. Also a growing number of clients will have home computers. The scope of this medium is immense and programmes have already been established that enable users to shop from home or to communicate with each other.

Therapists must determine which mediums they feel are appropriate to the client group they are using them with and which fall within the budgets or resources they have access to. Thought should also be given to how accessible the information is to members of ethnic groups and clients who have learning difficulties or are sensorily impaired. In the development of information it must be decided whether the information is to be used as a supplement to therapist led sessions or in isolation. If clients are to be given information without access to someone to discuss queries, the format and content should be very clear. While the provision of a booklet may convey information the use of group work can convey the same information but also provide levels of support.

The development of educational programmes is one way of conveying information to clients. Many of the educational approaches used by therapists tend to adopt either a behavioural or educational approach, thus having a defined structure and content. The effectiveness of these programmes in terms of conveying information has been demonstrated but the longer term effects in relation to functional ability or coping responses remains a matter for investigation.

A less formalized environment for conveying information and gaining support and advice is that of self-help groups.

SELF-HELP GROUPS

Recent years have seen the emergence of many self-help groups related to a wide and varied range of issues. They are seen as offering help and assistance from outside of 'the system' and so being less inhibited by bureaucracy and having the ability to reflect the voice of the people. It is also for this reason that the relationship between self-help groups and the statutory sector has not always been easy. There are many political issues, both with a capital and a small 'p' which surround the emergence of self-help, especially at a time when the services offered within the state system are receding and being criticized in many areas.

First, it is necessary to define what is meant by self-help, as the words tend to be used interchangeably with mutual aid, although these are two very different concepts. Self-help is fundamentally an egocentric concept epitomized by a capitalistic society. It relates the Victorian concept of the undeserving poor and is summarized in the following quotation from Samuel Smiles, 'The spirit of self-help is in the root of all genuine growth in the individual and exhibited in the lives of many constitutes the source of national vigour and strength. Help from without is often enfeebling in its effects but help from within invariably invigorates, whatever is done for men and classes to a certain extent takes away the stimulus and necessity of doing for themselves and where men are subjected to over guidance and over government the inevitable tendency is to render them comparatively helpless' (Smiles, 1958). Therefore the original concept of self-help does not equate, in many ways, with the general usage of the terminology today. Mutual aid, however, was seen as a co-operative process in the emergence of friendly societies and trade unions where people work together to assist each other. Both ideologies emerged from political roots and still carry political undertones with them. Most people refer to the underlying philosophy of mutual aid when they talk about self-help.

The re-emergence of self-help can be seen as a response to the bureaucratic welfare system; 'The welfare state tends to treat materials and practical problems rather than promote personal growth and a sense of personal worth. An established profession such as medicine has tended to treat symptoms and bodily illness rather than promote self-understanding, adjustment and a greater sense of wholeness. Self-help along with holistic medicine and a host of other new responses to problems has begun to fill a vacuum' (Landan North and Duddy, 1985). While this statement may be viewed by some as extreme in its view of a totally impersonal narrow profession it is apparent that such a large state run system cannot be as flexible and responsive to individual needs as locally based groups. Many would see self-help as complementing the services offered by the statutory sector.

A criticism of self-help is that it is attributing to the dismantling of the welfare system by taking on roles and providing services which should be available through the state system. While services are being provided by the voluntary sector there is a decreased demand on statutory services enabling them to negate responsibility for certain aspects of care, especially within the community.

Self-help has also been identified as a predominantly middle-class concept, which can be seen to be untrue in relation to co-operative societies and trade unions, and so only reflecting the voice of a small section of the population. The relationship with professionals can be tenuous in some circumstances especially when groups are seen to question aspects of their healthcare or management. 'Groups of people meeting in each other's home over tea or coffee pose no particular threat or concern. . . . However when a group of people having a particular problem come together to actively help themselves and others and attach the title self-help they are often viewed with suspicion and asked to explain the rationale for their existence' (Landan North and Duddy, 1985).

On a collective basis self-help groups are therefore seen as fulfilling both a social and a political role. The benefits for individual members are however more varied. Self-help groups are essentially groups of people who feel they have a common problem meeting together to exchange help and support and do something about the problem. Emphasis is on the idea of sharing and providing the opportunity to meet and learn from one another. This breaks away from the 'doctor–patient' relationship and emphasizes reciprocity.

For some members the groups provide a way in which they can contribute to solving some of their own problems and so feel more in control of their disease. As members become more involved in groups and have attended for a period of time they may gain a sense of being able to help other people by offering information or support. The organization of groups lends a degree of formality which emphasizes the difference between a self-help group and a group of friends, although some self-help groups also provide a social function for members outside of the meetings and friendships develop through contacts met at groups.

Groups also provide services beyond the group meetings, many Arthritis Care groups organize swimming sessions, some have welfare officers who visit clients at home and they also offer holiday accommodation at several places throughout the United Kingdom or organize group holidays abroad. Other groups concentrate on fund raising to help pay for research into a specific condition or campaign to increase public awareness regarding the condition, or political and social issues arising from it.

Self-help groups exist on two levels, the larger organizations tend to be national organizations with a head office and employed staff, producing literature on a national basis, such as Arthritis Care. These organizations usually have local groups and regional officers to provide support at a local level and encourage the development of new groups and initiatives.

Smaller local initiatives exist where a group of people have met and decided to start their own group, either because a larger group with which to affiliate does not exist, or, the one that does exist does not meet the needs as identified by that group who feel an alternative is necessary. An example of this may be a local group which consists of an older age group who meet on a purely social basis and a group of younger people with the same condition who want to find out more about their disease and actively campaign on specific issues. While the presenting condition of the clients is the same the needs as identified by the two groups are completely different. Local groups have the advantage over national organizations of being in touch with local needs. The needs of a head office based in London may reflect in no way the local needs of a group in the north of the country, whose priorities, needs and resources may be totally different.

The level of participation in group activities varies considerably. Some members are willing to adopt leadership roles while others prefer to stay in the background and attend meetings. Some common problems of self-help groups have been identified as:

1. getting people to adopt extra responsibility;
2. a high membership turnover making the running of groups and gaining stability difficult;
3. a low membership turnover making groups stale;
4. a shared problem bringing the group together invariably means that it functions under a handicap;
5. practicalities such as transport and finance (Richardson, 1984).

Non-participation in groups can be attributed to several factors, it may be a matter of choice not to join or it may be a lack of knowledge of the group's existence, problems of transport and finance can also inhibit membership as can the degree of support received from family. If a client is dependent upon her husband for transport to and from the meeting it is difficult to participate if he is against her attending. With thought and careful planning some of these problems can be overcome. The involvement of healthcare professionals with groups is an area which needs addressing, especially in relation to the role which professionals can play in supporting groups.

New groups are formed frequently from an individual who identifies an area of need and starts looking for help in meeting that need. If no form of help is available then advice may be sought about starting a self-help group. If a professional is approached at this stage consideration should be given as to whether to get involved or to refer the client to another agency more related to self-help initiatives than to statutory provision. In some areas Councils for Voluntary Services may exist or there may be Community Development Officers attached to Local Authorities. Such agencies have the skills to work alongside group members helping them to develop the skills necessary to start and maintain a self-help project. They will usually work alongside groups until the group is strong enough to run itself, providing help and support which is withdrawn gradually so that the group becomes self supporting.

If therapists become involved in groups, consideration should be given to the level of involvement and the way in which this can detract from the essence of self-help. If a high level of involvement is assumed it is difficult for group members to develop their own organizational skills and the group can become dependent upon the support of the 'professionals'. This is summed up in the following statement, 'professionals must learn to be enablers leading from behind. They should give support but not control, advise but not dictate, be available but not always around' (Landan, North and

Duddy, 1985). It is difficult when asked for help not to take over and take on responsibilities, especially when used to organizing and developing projects and perhaps knowing exactly where to go for assistance and knowing that the tasks could be completed in half the amount of time simply because you have ready access to the information and know ways around and through systems.

In addition to this founder members may still be feeling unsure of what they are meant to be doing and out of their depth and feel that a 'professional' will be able to help them overcome their problems. However if skills are going to be acquired by members, professionals must resist the temptation to become too involved, even though it may initially take longer to explain processes rather than carry them out. Support and advice should be given and practical assistance if necessary but preferably working alongside members and not actually taking on the work in isolation. Clients may feel initially dependent upon healthcare professionals as they are predominantly seen as service providers and clients as receivers. To reverse these roles could be threatening for clients whose expectations of professionals is one of taking the lead and may also be threatening to professionals who have been used to being in a controlling situation. The temptation to dominate, take on too many tasks and play an organizational role should be resisted.

Various guides and packages have been compiled to assist groups in establishing themselves. Once a group of people have been identified as wishing to develop a group many practical issues have to be considered. Decisions have to be taken as to the aims of the group, whether to provide information, provide support, organize campaigns, raise funds or plan social activities. The composition of the membership has to be identified as to whether it will comprise purely of people with the problems, or include family and other interested people. Thought also has to be given to the first meeting and a suitable venue identified. The accessibility of the venue can influence greatly the numbers of people getting to the meetings as can the availability of transport.

The content of the first meeting has to be identified, a format developed and chairperson elected. In order to maintain the momentum of the first meeting some thought should also be given to the second meeting so that the venue and topic can be announced and members feel a sense of continuity. Once these topics have been addressed the first meeting has to be publicized and potential members informed. While not being involved directly therapists can offer support to members trying to establish a group and contacts for advice and practical assistance. Advice may also be needed on ways of raising finance to contribute towards the cost of publicity, refreshments, rent for a venue, postage, etc.

Therapists have a role to play with established groups. Keeping a group running can demand a lot of energy from the organizers and they may need on-going support and advice. It is useful for them to know that there are some professionals who will offer support and information without taking over the group. As the membership of groups can change frequently on-going publicity is needed to attract new members. Therapists and clinicians have access to potential new members and can fulfil a valuable role by passing on information about groups and meetings. The other active role which can be played by therapists is that of taking meetings when asked or suggesting potential speakers or resources which may be of use.

Therapists can also utilize self-help groups as an invaluable source of information representing the real 'client voice'. In the development of services or programmes or the evaluation of work seeking representative client groups for opinions and comment can prove difficult. These groups rarely exist within the statutory sector and so have to be sought in the voluntary sector, primarily self-help groups.

Self-help groups can provide a valuable contribution to the management of a chronic disease providing a dimension of management which can not be offered by many healthcare professionals, the provision of information and support from the view point of a person with the condition. Therapists should endeavour to foster working relations with self-help groups and utilize the resources and services they can provide. Misunderstandings and threat are usually born through lack of communication and overprotection of identity, if these stumbling blocks can be overcome the value of working together can only add an extra dimension to the service offered to clients. The fostering of links and the active involvement of members of self-help groups in the work of departments of rheumatology should be encouraged.

COUNSELLING

The main emphasis of many therapeutic interventions in rheumatology are towards eleviating the physical manifestations of the disease, reducing symptoms and maintaining function. Previous chapters have considered the psychosocial impact of the disease and highlighted how these can also affect perception of, and in some instances induce, physical symptoms, and decrease levels of function. Personal and family relationships can also be affected and communication between family members can break down.

This section will consider the role of counselling in facilitating client's adjustment to living with a chronic disease and coping with crises if they occur. This will be addressed from the view point of the humanistic approach which is psychotherapeutic not psychoanalytical and is non-directive or client centred. This approach has been taken as it relates closely to the basis of occupational therapy.

Rogerian therapy is based upon an existential humanist approach and has influenced greatly counselling work. Rogerian theory emphasizes the wholeness of man, the responsibility of the individual for their life and their freedom to make choices. Humanist views believe in man's ability to understand himself and change or improve through his own efforts. Rogerian therapy is directed towards facilitating this process. This process involves the therapist in entering into a relationship of unconditional positive regard, being warm and supportive.

Through using skills such as active listening, physical attending, empathy and reflection, therapists aim to help clients identify and clarify their feelings. When using counselling skills the therapist is non-directive and never imposes views or opinions. The counsellor provides the environment in which clients can explore feelings or problems and arrive at their own definition of what they feel and the direction in which they wish to progress. This process is at the opposite end of the continuum to a behavioural approach which is directive and places the emphasis on the therapists status as 'professional' providing specific guidelines to follow and action to take.

The trend of psychotherapeutic interventions in clinical practice is directed predominantly towards crisis management rather than helping clients adjust to the significant changes in lifestyle, body image and role that can occur or work through the bereavement process associated with the losses they may be experiencing. Within clinical practice the onus is still more towards physical rather than psychological management. Some of the reasons for this include the basis of the medical model of care, the lack of validity of psychotherapeutic interventions and the amount of resources required to use these interventions.

The medical model of care is predominantly disease orientated with an emphasis on the physical component of disease and working towards curing or elieviating physical problems. A client presents with a problem which is taken on by the clinician, investigated and treated. The basis of counselling a client is that the therapist does not take on the client's problem but through the use of specific skills provides an environment which enables the client to address their own problem. The underlying philosophy of counselling is very different to a medical model of care.

Despite the increasing use of counselling in relation to rheumatoid disease little data exists which identifies the validity of this approach. Studies which have been conducted have failed to identify a statistically significant change in psychological parameters. This is an area in which research is proceeding confronted by the need to validate methods of intervention using criteria from a model of care which is in many ways opposed to the model being validated.

Embarking upon a process of individual counselling is a lengthy and labour intensive process. The allocation of therapist's time is a factor of consideration as resources become less available. It is essential that time allocation is considered before a client is taken on, as they cannot be abandoned after a few sessions if time becomes limited.

The initial period of counselling aims to explore and enable the client to clarify issues which they perceive as problems, the skills used are directed towards this and also establishing a therapeutic relationship with the client. An overview of the counselling process has been proposed as eight stages.

Stage 1 Meeting the client.
Stage 2 The discussion of surface issues.
Stage 3 Revelation of deeper issues.
Stage 4 Ownership of feelings and possible emotional release.
Stage 5 Generation of insight, the client's life is reviewed by them in a different light.
Stage 6 Problem-solving and future planning.
Stage 7 Action by the client.
Stage 8 Disengagement from the counselling relationship by the client (Burnard, 1989).

The main skills used in a counselling process are listening and attending, reflection, selective use of questions and summarizing. The distinction between hearing and listening is stated as 'Hearing involves the capacity to be aware of and receive sound. Listening involves not only receiving sounds but, as much as possible, accurately understanding their meaning. As such it entails hearing words, being sensitive to vocal cues, observing movements and taking into account the context of communication' (Nelson Jones, 1988). This involves paying attention not only to content but also to the tone of a person's voice, the pitch and the volume. Being party to a conversation in which you have not been listened to is a situation with which most people can identify and will be able to remember the frustration and anger felt. It is essential that the client is aware of the counsellor's attention and feels that they are being listened to. Becoming an active listener is a definite skill and involves the use not only of verbal skills but non-verbal communication as well. Attending is the skill of showing the client that they have your full attention and this is communicated by posture, gesture and other forms of non-verbal communication.

Reflection is probably the most widely recognized counselling skill as it is used to conjure up the stereotyped picture of a counsellor repeating parrot fashion what is being said. In fact it has several very specific uses. It is easy to relate on a personal level to the clarity that is gained by someone reflecting what you have said. Very often we think we have said something and the person listening hears something different. Reflection enables both the counsellor and client to check they are on the same line and talking about the same thing. Reflection also enables the client to hear, perhaps for the first time, their thoughts and feelings being verbalized. The process of verbalization can bring thoughts into perspective and help to identify if what is being said is really meant and clarify the feelings the client may be experiencing. While situations may be easy to explain sometimes the feelings attached to those experiences are more difficult to identify.

Questions should be open ended and relevant to what is being discussed and can be used to lead a client if they are experiencing difficulty in verbalizing a specific problem.

During this initial exploratory period the content of the interviews may be muddled, jump from one issue to another and bring out painful issues. It is necessary for the counsellor to summarize what has been said from time to time to try and make some links between what has been said and to clarify what is going on. The content often reflects the client's confusion at the early stages of the counselling process and as they feel more secure in the relationship they are able to move on to exploring issues in more depth.

The next phase of counselling focuses more on specific problems which have been highlighted in the exploratory period. These issues are looked at in detail to enable the counselling to move on to help the client identify possible ways of approaching the issues raised and dealing with them and the possible consequences of doing so. This enables clients to explore options within the safety of the relationship established with the counsellor and in some situations to try out possible responses with the counsellor before embarking upon facilitating change in their own situation.

The processes involved in counselling are described in many publications which provide exercises to carry out, either on an individual or group basis and references will be given. The use of these skills and the provision of space and time for the client to explore issues within a relatively safe environment is invaluable in assisting clients to adapt to change. The responsibility remains with the client and at no time does a counsellor take on the responsibility for the client's problems, they merely provide an environment in which problems can be identified, clarified and explored and responses learned and tried out.

Even if therapists feel that they do not have the time to become involved in counselling clients the development of counselling skills will help tremendously in their day to day work. The ability to be an active listener and to progress a conversation without imposing values or opinions is a skill which will contribute to the effectiveness of client/therapist relationships and provide the means to enable clients to explore the issues which are of importance to them.

Group counselling has also been used in relation to groups of clients with rheumatoid disease, the counsellor acting as group facilitator and using the dynamics of the group to identify and explore issues of relevance to that group. The structure and intention of such a group is different from a group of clients meeting as a self-help group, as a counselling group is usually closed, given some form of direction from the group leader (in relation to facilitating the group process) and runs for a set period of time.

This section has explored several settings in which therapists can be involved as a vehicle for communication. The structure of each setting is different, as is the role of the therapist in each. The aim of all of these settings is to provide an environment in which clients are active, if they want to be. They all focus on active participation and it must be remembered that for some clients this will not be appropriate. Some clients will wish to adopt a passive role and hand over the management of their disease to 'the professional'. Thought must be given as to whether this is due to a lack of skills and confidence on the client's behalf which could be developed, an entrenchment in the medical model of care which hands over all responsibility to the professional as this is their perceived role or a person who for various reasons has taken on a passive sick role in which they are happy.

Access to information, support and resources are essential components to coping with a chronic disease. The type of each will vary from client to client, some clients will find their support from friends in the club, others from a self-help group and others from within their own home. Some clients will want to find out as much information as possible about what they can be doing to help themselves, others will want to know very little.

The aim of a team should be to provide access to a variety of settings and approaches so that the needs of clients can be met on a broad spectrum. The active involvement of clients is dependent upon the attitudes of the therapists and clinicians they meet and the amount of information they have access to. The role of the team should be that of enabling clients and providing access to the services and resources which clients feel are important, supporting when necessary during times of need and then withdrawing to give clients the opportunity and space to develop their own skills. Empowering clients is an issue which to many clinicians is threatening, primarily as it means relinquishing power as a 'professional' but in rheumatology the onus has to be on ways in which clients can be empowered to help themselves.

The potential of occupational therapists to facilitate these approaches is immense as many of them are central to the underlying philosophy of the profession and form a significant component of therapist's training. While some of the concepts may be alien to the medical model of care and their potential not realized, as yet, therapists are ideally placed to introduce and implement such concepts, as a minimum, within their own clinical practice if not on a wider scale.

The general direction of healthcare is towards greater client involvement, a move which to some extent has been client led, and individual therapists must identify the most appropriate model of working for themselves, with the confidence however, to know that they have the skills and the hospital and community perspective to play a central role in a direction which is slowly becoming reality.

FURTHER READING

L. Ewles, I. Simnett (1985) *Promoting Health, A Practical Guide to Health Education*, John Wiley and Sons Ltd, London.

R. Nelson-Jones (1988) *Practical Counselling Skills*, 2nd edn, Cassell, London.

A. Richardson (1984) *Working with Self-Help Groups: A Guide for Professionals*, Bedford Square Press, London.

S. Rodmell, A. Watt (1986) *The Politics of Health Education, Raising the Issues*, Routledge and Kegan Paul, London.

W. Stewart (1985) *Counselling in Rehabilitation*, Croom Helm, London.

6

Adaptive techniques

Many different adaptive techniques are available to both therapists and clients to maintain independence and reduce the impact of rheumatoid disease on functional ability. These techniques can be used as components of self management programmes or on their own, in a group setting or on an individual basis. They are not only a means of maintaining function but also of enabling clients to achieve a sense of control over their disease. The ways in which rheumatoid disease can lead to feelings of helplessness have already been discussed and these techniques present practical ways in which a degree of control, no matter how small, can be achieved.

As techniques they are available to all clients to adopt. The aim of the therapist should be to present the principles in a way which is meaningful to the client and a way which seems realistic to incorporate in a daily routine without too much upheaval. By conveying principles the client is able to incorporate and adapt them as and when is appropriate. The time a client is in contact with any healthcare professional is fractional and clients should be given the information and the confidence which enables them to take a degree of responsibility in their care and be given the information necessary regarding how and when they may wish to seek the help of a 'professional'. The sharing of information is essential in the relationship of therapist and client and the role of therapist is one of 'enabling' and facilitating as well as in specific circumstances treating.

The aim of this chapter is to discuss some of these concepts and their application to the total management and life style of a client. The therapist and client together will need to identify the relevant concepts and work out realistic methods of application. As principles they remain guidelines and merely form a basis upon which to build. Collectively they comprise the principles of joint protection, which include energy conservation, as proposed by Joy Cordrey. The theoretical basis of these principles was an understanding of biomechanics, pathology of rheumatoid disease, the consequences of inflammation and anatomy (Cordery, 1965). This theoretical framework was developed into a set of principles which aimed to reduce the stress placed upon joints while carrying out activities of daily living in order to reduce pain, save energy and preserve the joint structures.

The principles comprise the following:

1. respect for pain;
2. balance between work and rest;
3. avoidance of positions of deformity;
4. maintenance of range of movement and muscle strength;
5. use of joints in their most stable position;
6. use of the strongest joints available to carryout an activity;
7. reduction of energy needed to complete an activity;
8. avoiding sustained positions or repetitive activities;
9. avoiding activities which cannot be stopped if they cause too much stress to joints or elicit high degrees of pain;
10. use of splints and assistive equipment to protect the joints (Melvin, 1977).

A brief explanation of these principles will be given, some will be considered in more depth in subsequent sections, followed by discussion of the dilemmas facing a therapist when presenting and using these principles.

Respect for pain

This relates to clients becoming aware of the types of pain they experience and differentiating between what is a normal level of background pain, which many clients experience each day, and what is pain caused by acute inflammation, or placing excessive force or strain on joints.

In most situations pain is seen as a warning signal of injury or illness and elicits a response to deal with the cause, which is usually avoidance and protection, however this situation differs with clients who experience chronic pain. The reverse occurs and clients need to develop coping strategies which place the pain in the background enabling activities of daily living to be carried out in spite of the pain being present. Pain clinics conduct courses aimed at helping clients to maintain levels of function and decrease pain-related behaviour which reinforces the intensity of pain felt.

The dilemma for clients with rheumatoid disease, however, is that they experience both acute and chronic pain and this is where an understanding of the nature of each is essential. Many clients experience a level of almost unremitting pain, if this pain were to be seen as a reason to rest joints and decrease functional activities movement would be lost, deformities develop and lifestyle would become very limited. However during an acute episode when joints are inflamed rest is needed and exercise should be limited in order to reduce the inflammation.

Clients, therefore, need to differentiate between acute and chronic pain and respond accordingly. This principle also relates to the point at which an activity is stopped due to pain. If, during an activity, pain becomes acute clients are advised to cease the activity as soon as possible. They should not continue until the level of pain becomes so unbearable that they have no choice other than to stop, as this is felt to increase inflammation and place undue stress on joint structures.

This principle relates to clients identifying the different types of pain they feel and acknowledging them.

1. What is an acceptable level of pain at which they must try to continue activities?
2. What is acute pain that is an indication that a joint is inflamed or has been subjected to too much activity or stress?
3. How can they respond to these different levels of pain within their lifestyle?

Balance between work and rest

This principle relates to the amount of rest and activity a client incorporates into their day and encompasses clients' concepts of each. The amounts will vary according to disease activity and therefore clients need to understand the principles of rest, activity and exercise and how the three are related. This principle is discussed in more detail under the heading of energy conservation.

Avoidance of positions of deformity

It is recommended that certain positions should be avoided as far as possible to decrease the development of deformities, for example placing pillows behind knees which encourages the development of flexion contractures. Clients should also be encouraged to lie flat on a bed, preferably on their stomach, to stretch the hip into full extension, if they are prone to the development of hip contractures. These principles also include the position of the hand during activities and the avoidance of positions that encourage the deformities of ulnar drift, swan neck, boutonniere, and subluxation of the MCP joints. Specific examples of the way in which this principle can be utilized are well documented in other publications. They mainly relate, with reference to hand function, to the use of alternative grips, the heel of the hand and the lateral edge of the palm as these are the strongest most stable parts of the hand and least vulnerable to stress. The use of two hands when lifting and the use of the forearm when carrying bags etc. as opposed to the hand are common examples.

Maintenance of range of movement and muscle strength

This principle is achieved through the use of a specific exercise programme designed to place each joint through a full range of movement to maintain movement, prevent the development of contractures and maintain muscle strength. Clients need to know the different types of exercise that can be carried out and how and when to up or down grade them according to disease activity. This principle will be discussed in more detail.

Use of each joint in its most stable position

The stability of joints can be compromised by destruction of the joint cartilage or bone or the lengthening of tendons or ligaments thus decreasing their stabilizing effect on the joint during movement. It was proposed that placing rotationary forces on joints such as the knees could increase this instability.

Use of the strongest joint to carry out an activity

This principle relates to distributing weight and stress to the largest joints during activities. So hips are used to push open doors rather than hand, palms are used to push rather than fingers etc.

Reduction of energy to carry out activities

This principle will be expanded in the energy conservation section and involves the use of energy saving equipment, the use of assistive equipment and forward planning.

Avoidance of holding sustained positions

Staying in one position for any length of time can lead to stiffness and pain on movement, clients will often relate how they dread getting up after they have been sitting for some time as they know how painful it will be. Therefore changes of position will help to decrease stiffness. Sustaining a static position can also be a cause of muscle fatigue and thus transmit stress to underlying ligaments and related structures.

Avoidance of activities which cannot be stopped

Starting an activity which cannot be stopped if pain occurs is placing a client in a position of having to continue through pain to complete the task. This principle relates to the planning of activities so that breaks can be incorporated if and when appropriate.

Use of assistive equipment and splints

In relation to joint protection the use of assistive equipment has been identified as:

1. supporting weakened joints, i.e. the use of walking aids;
2. to provide leverage to increase force while decreasing exertion;
3. to help maintain joints in the most stable anatomical position;
4. to extend reach when joints are limited in range of movement;
5. to avoid unnecessary use or strain, i.e. using a book rest when reading (Melvin, 1977).

One of the largest dilemmas facing therapists in the field of rheumatology is how they present these principles to clients and what basis this decision is taken from. While Cordrey has provided the theoretical basis for these principles this has not, as yet, been carried over into the clinical field. The main basis for using these principles initially was the reduction of deformity, but there remains a distinct lack of clinical data to substantiate the use of these principles on this basis. This is probably due to the enormous number of variables involved in such a long-term study. Some of these include the variability in the disease from client to client, the interpretation of each principle which leaves a great deal of scope for subjectivity, compliance over a long period of time and the large variation in clients' functional activities and lifestyles.

The variability of the disease from client to client is immense. In some clients destruction of joints occurs rapidly after onset necessitating joint replacement surgery within a relatively short space of time. Other clients can have the disease for years and while experiencing pain and other symptoms joint structures remain intact. It would therefore be difficult to ascribe the development or lack of development of deformity to the use of joint protection aside from the underlying disease process.

The interpretation of such concepts of rest and exercise and positions of deformity etc. are at the moment highly subjective. These terms would have to be defined much more precisely if they were to be the basis for an evaluative process.

The benefits of using joint protection in relation to the prevention of deformity, cannot be demonstrated over a short period of time. Compliance over a period of years would be difficult to sustain, especially as clients would not be receiving any immediate reinforcement.

The large variation in client's lifestyle and level and type of functional activity makes comparison between clients and control groups difficult. These are some of the problems which make the evaluation of joint protection in terms of prevention of deformity difficult. It has been proposed that the objective of joint protection be redefined as 'pain relief, reduction of internal and external stress to the joint, and decreasing inflammation within the patient's life-style. Success in obtaining these objectives should be clinically evident', and two possible definitions of joint protection proposed as being either in relation to 'preservation of structural components in a biomechanical frame of reference, with a cause effect relationship-slowing progression of joint deterioration' or as 'the enhancement of joint utilization in a functional sense – by avoiding pain and increasing function' (Shapiro-Slonaker, 1984).

One phrase which should be reiterated is 'within the patient's lifestyle'. Therapists must ask themselves what is the realistic level of use of these principles? It may be that they are used primarily during periods of exacerbation because this is the time at which pain and fatigue are at their worst and it seems more appropriate. In some environments, like work, clients may have little control over the way in which they work, the amount of rest they can take or the ability to cease an activity if it becomes painful. The choice of how these principles are used is always the clients and therapists should respect this fact and present joint protection in a way which is meaningful and realistic to each client.

The phrase 'joint protection' is in itself misleading as it can be seen to imply protecting joints from pain. While this is fundamental to the principles some of them equally refer to overcoming the body's natural protectiveness toward noxious stimuli. If a joint is painful the natural inclination is not to move it. While in some situations this is correct in others it can have dire consequences, leading to muscle weakness, the development of contractures, loss of function and more pain. The natural inclination to flex a joint when in pain is another example, if a person has painful knees the pain can be reduced by flexing the knee, yet while in the short term pain relief may be gained in the long term flexion deformities may develop. Clients will often say how during periods of exacerbation the only comfortable posture to adopt is a flexed one, not only of knees, but also of upper limbs with rounded shoulders, flexed fingers and bent elbows. Thus, some of these principles aim to overcome the long-term consequences of the body's natural reaction and method of protection.

Before embarking upon the process of teaching clients the principles of joint protection therapists need to consider carefully the way in which they will present them. Is it appropriate to present information on the basis that it is a means of preventing the onset of deformity when the basis for this is as yet not at all clear? In the long term it is unlikely that the original therapist will be present to answer the questions of clients who have developed deformity inspite of using joint protection principles and clients may be left wondering what they have done wrong.

The reduction of pain and increase of function through using these principles can, however, be seen immediately. Clients will receive quick feedback as to whether using energy conservation techniques enables them to do more, or whether the use of assistive equipment elicits less pain when performing an activity. Whichever interpretation therapists choose there is still the responsibility to evaluate its basis. Data is needed in relation to the effectiveness of the principles of joint protection whether in relation to decreasing deformity, pain or internal or external stress on joints during activity, otherwise the basis for asking clients to fundamentally change their life-style will always remain questionable, and how can therapists answer with any conviction the client who asks 'why should I do this?' or the clinician who asks 'why should I refer clients to you to be taught joint protection?' Some of these principles will now be considered in more detail.

ENERGY CONSERVATION

Fatigue and lack of energy are expressed frequently as having a major impact on a person's functional ability. This symptom may not, initially, be associated by the client with the disease process as the articular manifestations of the disease are more widely recognized by clients than the systemic. Fatigue and lack of energy can be the expression of either a physical or psychological state or a combination of both.

The disease process can cause fatigue often associated with an increase in disease activity as more energy is expended in dealing with the inflammatory response. Anaemia may also lead to depleted energy levels as can the decreased ability of weak muscles to carry out daily activities. Pain and stiffness frequently lead to loss of sleep which over a period of time can prove as debilitating as articular manifestations, and coping with chronic pain can be debilitating in itself.

In relation to stress, anxiety and depression, fatigue can be viewed as either a cause or a symptom. Constantly feeling tired and lacking in energy can lead to a decrease in functional ability and feeling of frustration and a sense of failure which may lead to depression. Alternatively a client undergoing a period of reactive or endogenous depression may be experiencing fatigue as a symptom of that depression.

As a symptom there are several ways in which clients can adapt their lifestyle to incorporate energy conservation into a daily routine and thus lessen the impact of decreased energy on function, hopefully avoiding the frustration and feelings of loss of control which can be associated with not having the energy to fulfil previous roles. The term energy conservation can be misleading to clients because it implies saving energy. It should be emphasized that this is not the object but rather making the most of the energy available and ensuring that it is used effectively.

The main principles of energy conservation relate to:

1. pacing;
2. forward planning;
3. work simplification.

PACING

Pacing refers to the use of rest, exercise and activity and their relationship to each other. The basis of communicating this concept lies, initially in establishing a client's understanding of each. Rest can be perceived as anything from reading to gardening, i.e. anything which is not work. Activity and exercise are often combined so that clients will perceive doing activities of daily living as exercise and therefore see no need to carry out a regular programme of exercise. By understanding the role of each of these three concepts clients will be able to use them to achieve a balance according to their varying needs and disease activity. The proportion of each will vary according to disease activity and to some extent the client's previous use of each before disease onset. Some people find sitting down and relaxing very difficult, preferring to be on the move. To suddenly incorporate rest into such a life-style can be difficult.

Rest may be applied to one specific joint, being local, the whole body, often called systemic, and psychological which includes relaxation. Local rest refers to the resting of a specific joint due to an increase in inflammation. It is usually achieved by the use of splints such as resting splints for the hands and wrists. Systemic rest refers to total body rest and this is sometimes used during periods of exacerbation when a client is admitted to a unit for a period of bed rest. The interpretation and use of bed rest varies from unit to unit. In some instances it will mean complete rest with clients being wheeled to the toilet for a period of, on average seven to ten days, while in others it will mean alternating between bed and chair with some degree of mobility allowed. Even during periods of complete rest some degree of exercise will be carried out in the form of passive exercise or gentle range of movement exercise. Emotional rest refers to relaxation of the mind. A person may be physically resting but emotionally active thinking of the tasks which need to be completed next or feeling guilty about sitting down in the middle of the day. If the mind is active and stressed muscles will be tense and the benefits of rest decreased. Relaxation can be used to cope with the symptoms of stress and anxiety and also as a means of coping with pain. Relaxation will be discussed in more detail.

The need to rest throughout the day is often a need which elicits feelings of guilt and failure. Sitting down can be regarded as 'giving in'. Therapists need to convey the positive aspects of rest which are primarily that when used correctly it enables more to be achieved by the end of the day, and that during periods of inflammation joints need to be rested to help decrease the inflammation. The usual way to complete a day's activity is to commence in the morning and work through until the tasks are completed with perhaps a break for lunch and coffee. A client will often try to retain this pattern of work and complete tasks even though this may lead to joint pain. Once a joint has been worked enough to elicit pain an activity has to be stopped and rest is enforced. Rest should be used before pain becomes so unbearable that activity is stopped. Short and frequent rests may increase functional activity.

Specific exercise programmes will usually be provided by physiotherapists in order to maintain or increase muscle strength and range of movement and prevent or correct deformities. However these must be incorporated into the daily routine and used in conjunction with rest and activity. Clients should be taught the rationale behind the programmes as well as the specific exercises.

Generalizations like 'exercise each day' or 'here is a list of exercises' serve little purpose in relation to a condition where disease activity is so variable and programmes need to be up or down graded frequently. If clients are given the information regarding the different types of exercise and their use then they will be able to adapt them to their varying needs.

The most common types of exercise used in relation to rheumatoid disease are isometric exercises and range of movement exercises. Isometrics are used frequently during periods of exacerbation as they entail muscular contractions without movement of the joint, thus helping to maintain muscle strength. Range of movement exercises are used to place specific joints through their full range of movement and may be passive or active.

It is essential to distinguish between exercise and activity as clients often see activity as a substitute for exercise. Daily activities rarely place all joints through a full range of movement especially if the working environment has been organized to simplify work. Many daily activities are carried out within an inner- to mid-range of movement and a good example of how movement can be lost by use purely within a functional range is the elbow joint. The number of times a day in which full elbow extension is achieved in relation to activities is negligible and many clients present with limitation in elbow extension. Loss of movement only usually becomes apparent to clients when function is affected and by this time movement may have been permanently lost.

It should not be assumed that any of us know what the full range of movement is for each of our joints and that limitations would be noticed. If clients are shown what their full range of movement is and how to monitor it then they will be in a better position to identify when limitations occur and seek help before contractures develop. Ways of grading exercises should also be taught so that programmes can be varied according to disease activity. During periods of remission exercises may be increased whereas during periods of exacerbation a family member may be required to assist in a passive range of movement.

Physiotherapists will work with clients when specific interventions such as passive stretching, or ultrasound are required but basic information regarding exercise should be available if clients are to carry out their own programmes.

Activity can refer to a whole spectrum of occupation ranging from sitting at a desk typing to completing a physically arduous task. In relation to pacing, clients are being asked to examine the type of activities in which they engage and identify ways of arranging the activities so that demanding tasks are alternated with less demanding activity. If possible tasks requiring repetitive movements should be interspersed with either a break or an activity which uses other joints and muscle groups balancing the work so that no one joint or muscle group is being asked to sustain activity in a repetitive manner for any length of time. It is this factor which sometimes leads to problems in employment situations where clients may be working on a production line continually carrying out repetitive movements with few breaks or opportunities to change position. Activities which require prolonged grip or repetitive movements can lead to an increase in pain and inflammation.

One example of this was a client who was working on a production line operating a machine to place the metal button on jeans. The work was repetitive in relation to upper limb function, sitting position and the trunk rotation needed to pass the garment on to the next person. There was no control over work rate, as she was part of a production line, and the garment, being denim, was heavy. It became necessary to consider alternative work and the employer allocated her to a different activity in the factory which was less arduous. Alternating periods of high activity with periods of rest may increase a client's functional ability, if the environment in which the client is functioning allows this.

The concept of pacing refers to the way in which rest, exercise and activity are used in relation to each other, disease activity and the functional requirements of a client. The optimum use of them is seen more often when a client has control over the content and structure of their day. In an employment situation it may appear difficult to incorporate periods of rest or to alternate activities. In some employment situations employers are prepared to adopt a flexible attitude to the way in which an employee uses their time allowing them to restructure their day to suit their needs, within a realistic structure. However, it is not always possible especially if the working environment is dictated by production lines where the next person's work is dependent upon every component of the process functioning in a set manner. Another client who presented with work-related problems was working for a local authority as part of a team laying kerb stones. The work was physically very demanding, obviously outdoors and the team were paid according to the footage of kerbstone laid. The incentive therefore placed more pressure on the client to keep up with his colleagues as any variation in his work not only slowed the team down but also directly affected their wage packets. In these situations the ability to use such principles can seem tantalizing to someone who has little control over their level of activity, but is faced with the choice of maintaining work or facing unemployment, and therapists are confronted with the problem of compromising principles to adjust to the reality of life.

FORWARD PLANNING

The principles of forward planning will not appear strange to anyone who has participated in a time management course. They are as useful to therapists with a large case load as to clients with rheumatoid disease. Forward planning and time management apply to both work and leisure. The way in which activities are carried out throughout the day or week is often, for most people, at best a question of meeting certain demands and needs as and when they occur with no formal statement of intent, and at worst a series of crisis management. For a person with limited energy and changing levels of function the way in which time is managed becomes more important and the setting of priorities essential.

The principles of forward planning can be conveyed in a practical and meaningful way for most clients. Most of us can relate to never having the time to complete all that we wanted to or leaving important tasks to the last moment and then placing ourselves in a crisis situation!

A starting point from which to convey this concept is to ask clients to write a record of what they have done for several days and to also include everything that they had to leave due to pain or stiffness. This record will then provide a basis for looking at how the client is at present using their time and energy and whether or not they are achieving a balance of work, rest and activity.

It then becomes possible to divide the activities into various categories such as work-related, leisure, rest, family, and exercise. Clients will then be able to see how much time is apportioned to each aspect of their life and how this relates to their present priorities. Frequently clients may be placing a large amount of time in maintaining employment or completing specific tasks to maintain independence. This is often at the cost of time spent with the family or in leisure activities. It may well be that the total amount of time allocated to different types of activity has not been considered previously and the imbalance of activity not perceived. At certain stages in disease progress, usually ones of transition to adapting to a loss of function, or during periods of exacerbation, this imbalance may reflect the client's priority as they try to maintain or regain levels of function, needing to devote more time to one aspect of their life, or purely that more time is needed to carry out activities.

The use of rest and exercise can also be identified and at what times they occur. If a person is always resting at the end of the day with no further periods of activity this may be an indication that they are continuing to work until levels of pain or fatigue are so great that they have to stop. Having identified a pattern of activity it then becomes possible to work with the client to identify ways of planning more effective use of their time to incorporate periods of rest and exercise and ensure that effective use is made of time allocated for activities.

Daily 'to do' lists will be familiar to those who use forward planning in their work. At the beginning of the day clients are asked to write a list of all that they need to do during that day. This is a way of using time before morning stiffness has worn off when many clients tend to sit and loosen up. This list should include both work and leisure activities. Having compiled the list the activities are then prioritized in order of importance. Initially the activities are graded

115

with an A, B, or C. then working through the list of As each activity is given a number, so A1 becomes the most important task to complete and should be completed first.

This method of working ensures that priorities are carried out and that clients are not placing themselves in the position of being tired and having to push themselves to complete activities which have to be done that day. As the activities become less important it becomes easier to leave them to the next day. Activities can be carried over from one day to the next and their priority reassessed.

Forward planning also enables periods of predicted activity to be incorporated into a week with allowances for more rest. If clients know that they have been invited out or are expecting to have to complete a demanding task they can allow periods of rest either before or after the activity.

Forward planning is the practical means by which pacing is incorporated into a daily schedule by identifying priorities and ways of organizing time to incorporate all the necessary elements of a day.

WORK SIMPLIFICATION

This is based upon the use of activity analysis and ergonomics and aims to increase the efficiency with which specific activities are carried out. Working environments, especially in the home, may not be laid out in the most efficient way. By asking a client to map out the distances walked while carrying out a simple task like making a cup of tea a visual picture of working practice can be made. From this it may be possible to discuss ways in which changes can be made to decrease unnecessary activity.

While many of the principles used seem common sense it is often these which are overlooked and yet they are in many cases, the most relevant and applicable. They include the following:

1. the organization of working environments giving consideration to correct working heights, position of work and the accessibility of frequently used items;
2. the type of equipment being used i.e. weight, size and ease of use;
3. the use of labour saving equipment;
4. saving repeated journeys by organizing such things as what needs to be taken up and down stairs and doing it in one trip;
5. breaking activities down into smaller constituents;
6. delegating tasks to other family members.

Delegation, although purported to be the art of good management, is often one of the most difficult things to do, whether associated with a colleague or family member. Asking for assistance can be seen as giving in or admitting failure or can be the cause of guilt or embarrassment. The higher the personal value ascribed to the activity the more difficult it becomes to delegate to someone else or to seek assistance with. Communication between family members will allow the personal space to complete highly valued tasks while absorbing the more routine and less important ones.

Spending time with clients discussing their present lifestyle and how they carry out activities will provide a clearer idea of factors which may be contributing towards the levels of fatigue they may be experiencing. Energy conservation is a misleading term because it implies saving energy and does not convey the positive motive behind it which is to maximize the use of energy to achieve priorities and maintain function. It incorporates the treatment modalities of rest and exercise alongside activities of daily living and provides an active way in which clients can begin to explore ways of adjusting lifestyles to attain goals.

THE USE OF ASSISTIVE EQUIPMENT

The use of assistive equipment is considered when function is limited by the effects of an impairment. It may be introduced as a short-term measure following joint replacement surgery to limit extremes of movement temporarily in order to protect the new joint or long-term when the physical capacity to carry out an activity is compromised. The range of equipment available to maintain functional ability has never been greater. Markets for products extend internationally giving access to equipment previously not available. The increase in competition has led manufacturers to pay more attention to the needs of clients and therapists when developing a product and to consider the aesthetics of the product alongside design and safety factors. For many clients the greatest constraint on access to equipment is financial. With local authority budgets coming under closer scrutiny access to therapists and equipment is limited and often compromised by financial constraints placing limitations on what can be provided through the statutory sector. While more clients are deciding to purchase their own equipment the cost can in many instances be prohibitive.

Many factors need to be considered when identifying the

appropriate piece of equipment for the client, these factors are physical, psychological, social and environmental. The process of assessment for equipment can be broken down into the following stages.

1. Identify the clients' needs.
2. Consider physical, psychological, social and environmental factors which may influence choice.
3. Consider other factors which may influence choice, i.e. funding or policies.
4. Identify equipment which may be appropriate and sources of provision.
5. Explain rationale behind the choice of equipment to client and, if appropriate, their family.
6. Instruct in the use of equipment.
7. Re-evaluate after a period of use.

The provision of equipment may, for a therapist, be a matter of routine but for clients may be seen as an indication of the progression of the disease and a deterioration in their ability to carry out fundamental activities. Some clients see the use of equipment as giving in and will try to carry on for as long as possible without using it. Another barrier which needs to be overcome by many clients before accepting equipment into their homes is the look of equipment and the visual indication this gives to visitors of a client's limitation.

IDENTIFYING CLIENTS' NEEDS

Having carried out a functional assessment, areas of limitation will have been identified. The first decision is whether the limitation is a problem to the client and how much of a problem they themselves perceive it to be. Assessment may have highlighted a client's inability to get in and out of the bath but this does not automatically mean that this is a problem to the client. They may be happy washing at the sink or having the bath attendant in to assist them. In some cases the physical or social contact that assistance with activities of daily living brings is more important than the independence of completing an activity without assistance. The priority given to aspects of function by the client may differ from that of the therapist. If several areas of need have been identified the client's priorities associated with each area must be identified.

Physical, psychological and environmental factors influencing choice

Physical factors which contribute to a decrease in function are:

- pain;
- loss of movement;
- fatigue;
- weakness;
- stiffness;
- deformity.

Consideration should be given to the source of pain, movements which elicit it or prevent it and any variation which may occur. Liaison is needed with other team members to ascertain whether other interventions have been tried or whether they are indicated. As has already been discussed some positions which decrease pain are contraindicated as they can lead to deformity, therapists must be conscious of this. An example of this is clients who find sleep difficult due to pain and find a flexed posture comfortable to sleep in. Electric beds enable a posture of flexed hips and knees to be assumed all night but may be contraindicated due to the possible development of hip and knee contractures.

The amount of stress placed on joints while using assistive equipment should be considered also as this may lead to increased pain. This can be illustrated with the use of bathboards and seats. While these may assist a client to transfer into the bath the use of this equipment places a great deal of strain on upper limbs which can cause pain. Rope ladders used to help people to sit up in bed can increase strain on the upper limbs leading to pain.

Loss of movement may be as a result of joint destruction, pain, deformities and contractures. Liaison is again essential to ensure that equipment is not compensating for movement which could be regained with a course of physiotherapy. A client may be on a waiting list to undergo joint replacement surgery and this may have a bearing on the equipment provided. A therapist may feel that it is advisable to provide a temporary solution to the problem and reassess the client's functional ability post-surgery. This dilemma is a difficult one to address. A person with degenerative arthritis may have single joint involvement and there may be a dramatic improvement in their functional ability post-operatively. A person with multiple joint involvement may see little change in their functional ability post-operatively but pain levels may be reduced significantly. Few functional activities utilize only one joint and the completion of functional activities may still be compromised by limitation and pain in other joints.

If fatigue is a major cause of limitation energy conservation and pacing may improve function. However the provision of some equipment may be indicated to enable clients to utilize the principles of energy conservation, such as perching stools or trolleys.

Weakness is a major limiting factor in relation to hand function, where reduced grip compromises function, and also in relation to mobility.

Stiffness can lead to a fluctuation in functional ability, especially in relation to the morning. Clients will often have to wait for stiffness to wear off before they can begin to carry out activities. It can also inhibit function if a client has been maintaining one position for any period of time so that transfers can become more difficult the longer a person is seated.

The development of contractures can limit function in relation to many aspects of activities of daily living. If these contractures are reversible function may improve following therapy. If deformities are permanent they may influence the choice of equipment. Clients who have developed flexion contractures of hips and knees are often unable to use many of the types of bath aids available as they do not accommodate such limitations in movement. Deformities of the hand may limit finger extension and the size of some kitchen aids may be too large to grip, or alternatively limited flexion may mean that handles are too small.

The variability of the physical symptoms of rheumatoid disease should also be considered. The difference between a client's functional ability on a good day and a bad day can be immense. In relation to an activity such as bathing, a client may, during a period of remission, be able to bathe independently using a bath board and seat and yet during a period of exacerbation require something which offers a much greater degree of assistance. For this reason some clients prefer equipment which is portable, so that during periods of remission it can be put away and is not obvious or intrusive. Therapists must be aware of the possible adverse effect of providing equipment which supplements movement which could be regained or places the client in positions which may lead to the development of deformity.

Psychosocial factors which influence the choice of equipment include the client's perception of their need, their acceptance of their disability and their attitude to the use of equipment. If a client has not accepted their disability and is denying the effects of the disease it is unlikely that they will accept the need for assistive equipment to be used. As it is so material it is difficult to deny its function and the use of such equipment means an acceptance of some limitation. For many clients the use of equipment is usually considered when the completion of activities independently becomes more important than incorporating the use of equipment into the self-concept or levels of pain become intolerable.

Clients seem to perceive a hierarchy of equipment so that, initially, the use of small equipment to help with food preparation is perceived as providing help whereas the use of a larger piece of equipment in the bathroom is not accepted as it is seen as an indication of being in need of more assistance and being labelled as disabled. Therapists are frequently told, 'I haven't got to that stage yet but it is reassuring to know what is available'.

Clients will often have a perception of how their need can be met before they meet a therapist and have expectations of how these problems are to be overcome. Community therapists often relate how they are constantly being asked for showers to be installed and receiving requests for specific equipment. It must be remembered that clients will very infrequently have a great knowledge of exactly what equipment is available and it is logical to request a shower if climbing in and out of the bath is difficult. This does not necessarily reflect a dogmatism on the client's behalf but a lack of information regarding all the options available.

It is wrong to assume that clients want to achieve independence in all aspects of daily living; some may be happy receiving assistance. This is when the involvement of family or carers becomes important. If both the client and carer are happy giving and receiving assistance and when options are explained still wish to continue as before, there is little point in spending time and resources in trying to increase independence. A client with a young family may have a routine worked out whereby her husband gets her dressed and washed in the morning and gets the children ready for school. This family may have worked out their own routine which suits their lifestyle and needs.

Problems do arise, however, when a client has adopted a dependent role and expects their partner to provide a level of assistance which they are not able or prepared to offer. Therapists can then be faced with a client who is refusing to accept the use of equipment because they perceive their carer as fulfilling the function and a carer who, in some situations, is being expected to provide an unrealistic level of support. In this situation communication between partners is essential if assistance is ever going to be provided. So many factors can contribute to such a situation including denial on the behalf of the client as to the level of demand they are making, apprehension about accepting help from other people, anger and frustration that they have limitations and on the carer's behalf guilt about not fulfilling a caring role and possibly about being healthy and independent. In this situation it is essential that both partners begin to communicate and understand each others point of view.

Clients' attitudes towards equipment will also influence its use. Some of the compromises clients are asked to make would be difficult for most of us to accept. If a client is unable to get upstairs to the bathroom they may have to bring their bed downstairs and use a commode. This can be embarrassing for the client who is dependent upon someone else to empty it and also in some situations for other members of the family. One client recounted her obvious distress when her teenage son told her that he was too embarrassed to bring his friends home because the living room was now used as a bedroom and 'not like other peoples' homes'. While it is easy to say that this is a stage that teenagers go through it helped neither the mother or her son. The criteria for provision of equipment or housing adaptations should be broad enough to include social as well as physical factors.

Consideration should also be given to the type of assistance another member of the family is being asked to provide and whether this is acceptable to both the client and the carer. An example of this is in relation to bathing. Husbands and wives have certainly been encountered who have never seen each other in the bath and would find the situation acutely embarrassing if asked to do so. Assumptions and valued judgements should never be made about the level or type of assistance family members are prepared to give. In some families the level of care can be intimate and cause no embarrassment whatsoever but this should not be taken for granted. The needs of other family members should be taken into account alongside those of the clients and may influence choice of equipment, especially if carers have some form of limitation in their ability to offer assistance. A carer with back problems may not be able to lift some of the bath aids provided out of the bath.

If a client is reliant upon the assistance of carers from outside the family these carers should be familiar with the safe and proper use of the equipment. A classical example of this is the use of hoisting equipment. The carers going into a client's home may change regularly, especially over holiday periods, and not all carers may be familiar with the use of equipment. While therapists cannot ensure that every person using the equipment will be familiar with it key people should be identified and taught how to use it. This factor encroaches upon the topic of training of community care staff in the use of equipment and is a training commitment in which many therapists are involved.

Environmental factors such as, size and layout of room, width of doorways, structure of walls and floor and accessibility to power can effect the choice of equipment. The type of environment in which the equipment is going to be used will also play a part. It may be a place of work as well as home and therefore the suitability for use in both environments must be considered alongside portability.

Other factors influencing choice

While therapists may identify a piece of equipment which is appropriate for the client other factors may limit the supply of it to the client. In a world where budgets were limitless there would be no constraint other than the need of the client. However supply of equipment through the statutory sector is dependent upon budget. The range of equipment available to the client if they choose to purchase privately is much greater. This can be shown in relation to wheelchairs where the Disablement Services Authority provides an adequate range of wheelchairs but the style, fabrication and performance of chairs purchased privately is very different. It is sometimes possible to gain assistance with funding for equipment via charities, trusts and, in relation to employment through the Disablement Advisory Service.

Identifying equipment

As the range of equipment available increases therapists rely more on information networks to keep them up to date with new products. A knowledge of the standard provision via the statutory sector is essential, as this is usually the starting place for provision. If the standard equipment range does not meet the needs of the client then therapists need to identify alternatives. Information networks regarding equipment are published by the Disabled Living Foundation in the form of equipment lists and another resource is the Equipment for Disabled People series of books. The DHSS also publish equipment evaluations where a range of a category of equipment is given to clients and reports compiled as to how the clients compared the different pieces of equipment and what advantages and disadvantages had been identified.

At a local level Disabled Living Centres have a display of equipment for clients and therapists in use and an extensive back-up of literature. This resource is excellent for clients wishing to purchase equipment privately. Disabled Living Centres are staffed, usually by occupational or physiotherapists and are open on an appointment basis for clients to call in. Clients are able to receive independent advice about equipment and also use the equipment to see if it is appropriate. The range of equipment displayed will vary according to the size of the centre but equipment which is not on display can usually be obtained for a specific assessment. Centres are involved frequently in holding study days and seminars related to equipment and usually have excellent relationships with the supplier and manufacturers of equipment.

COMMON FUNCTIONAL PROBLEMS

Seating

The main problems encountered in relation to seating are:

- Transfers – pain, stiffness and loss of movement;
- Comfort – pain, stiffness, altered posture, nodules.

Considerations

- the possibility of adapting existing chair;
- the amount of assistance needed to rise, will extra height be enough is spring assistance needed or a motorized chair raise;
- the dimensions required, height, depth, width of seat, length of back;
- accommodation of any deformity, scoliosis, flexion contractures etc.;
- if mechanical, the method of control and ease of use of controls.

Range of equipment

Adapting existing chair Clients who have problems in rising from a chair will try frequently to increase the height by placing several cushions on the seat. While this achieves a heightened seat it completely alters the dimension of the seat raising the seat and usually making the arms too low to rest on. If the chair offered any lumbar support this will now be in the wrong place and support for the head and neck may also be lost. It is more appropriate to raise the chair from the base rather than the seat.

Chair raisers can be purchased which heighten the chair either by inserting the legs into a sleeve or by replacing castors with screw-in legs. A platform can also be built which raises the chair the required height and into which the castors sink to avoid slipping when the client sits down. If a seat sags placing a piece of hard board under the cushion may provide extra support.

Neck cushions can be made or purchased to provide support to painful necks. Lumbar cushions can prove useful to people with low back pain, these are usually in the form of foam wedges or inflatable cushions.

Purchasing new chairs When assisting a client in choosing an appropriate seat, factors to consider include the height, width and depth of the seat, the amount of back support provided, the height of the back, angle of the seat, padding and type of armrest. Chairs can be too high as well as too low. Clients are often tempted to buy a seat which is high and therefore easy to rise from. Feet should be able to reach the floor easily. A chair which is too high will not support ankles and lead to increased pressure on the thighs, or slipping down the seat. It is worth checking before commencing assessment that the client is wearing the type of footwear they would normally be wearing in the house. If the client is assessed in shoes with a two inch heel and normally wears flat shoes around the house the assessment will be incorrect.

The front edge of the seat should not dig into the back of a client's knees. Some chairs provide very little back or head support. If a person has cervical involvement they should not have to extend their neck to gain support. The most comfortable seat is not necessarily one with a horizontal seat. A seat angle of about six degrees actually prevents slipping and slumping in the seat by slightly flexing the hips. If a client has nodules on their elbows it is more comfortable if the armrests are padded rather than wooden.

125

A good grip on the end of the armrest will also assist in transferring. There are a wide variety of chairs on the market, many of which are made to specific dimensions and some of which can be made to the requirements of the individual client.

Self-lift seats If, having tried a chair which is the correct height, the client still has difficulty in transferring it will be necessary to consider an assistive mechanism. Self-lift chairs provide a sprung seat which assists the client to stand. It is necessary to assess the seat the same way as above, ensuring the dimensions are correct and then to assess the strength of spring needed. Some chairs are adjusted by adding or removing springs from the seat, others have gauges which can be altered and some are set at the time of purchase by the manufacturer. The spring is set according to the client's weight. When they are seated the back of the seat should be flat. If the seat is not flat the spring is too heavy and should be decreased. If when the client goes to stand they feel they are getting no assistance the spring could be increased.

Some self-lift seats have a locking mechanism so that the seat remains flat until the mechanism is released. This ensures that if a client is sitting and, for example, reaches forward to pick something up from the floor the seat does not move and push them forward. While this extra safety factor is beneficial the mechanisms are often too stiff for clients with weak grip to operate.

Motorized chair An increasing number of electrically-operated chairs are available. The functions they offer vary from the seat unit raising, the whole chair raising so that back support is provided, to reclining as well. The most flexible chair has three independent motors which can work in isolation. Most chairs recline in one action, so that as the feet raise the back reclines. A client who spends a large amount of time in a chair may not always want to recline fully. There may be occasions when they wish to raise their feet but also sit up to eat or watch television or talk to someone. The flexibility of independent motors allows this.

Clients frequently request a reclining chair and find that they do not have the upper limb strength to operate the mechanism. Certain models of recliners can be motorized so that they recline electrically. These chairs can also offer the option of assisting in standing if this is needed. A guide to choosing a chair is published by the Arthritis and Rheumatism Council which covers the range of chair available.

Bathing

The main problems relate to:

- Transfers;
- Personal hygiene;
- Comfort.

Considerations

- client's functional ability;
- type of bath, size and layout of bathroom;
- availability of assistance;
- requirements of other family members;
- presence of nodules or leg ulcers;
- post-operative precautions.

A wide range of equipment is available to assist clients and their carers in relation to bathing. The complexity of use ranges from a fundamental board and seat to an overhead hoist used in combination with slings. While the prime concern is to enable the client to transfer independently or to assist the carers in transferring the client, thought should also be given to other aspects of personal hygiene. If a client is provided with equipment which enables them to transfer independently but they are unable to undress or wash themselves they will still not have achieved independence in bathing.

The existence of leg ulcers may mean that, at least until the ulcer has healed, the client should not be bathing and this should be checked with the nurse who is responsible for the dressing regime. A client with sacral nodules may find sitting on the hard surface of a bath or bathing equipment very uncomfortable and need some form of cushioning to enable them to sit down in comfort.

If a client has undergone a total hip arthroplasty specific precautions may be indicated post-operatively. Some surgeons advise their clients not to get in and out of the bath for twelve weeks post-operatively. This regime will vary however and should be clarified with the appropriate surgeons.

Bathboards and seats Bathboards and seats are usually the first consideration for therapists. The range on the market varies considerably in materials and fixing mechanism but all basically fulfil the same function. Boards are used frequently to assist clients in getting into the bath, by sitting on the board and swinging legs over into the bath. Painful metatarsal heads can make standing on the floor in bare feet painful and this can affect balance, therefore if clients can transfer sitting down they may experience less pain and be more stable.

Boards are used frequently in combination with an overbath shower enabling clients to shower seated. Boards which rest upon the top of the bath however can cause some problems as tucking the shower curtain inside the bath is difficult. Some boards and seats can be wall mounted enabling shower curtains to hang normally but, this is dependent upon the structure of the wall and the weight of the client. Boards should always be fitted securely to prevent slippage when the client transfers.

Seats vary in design and style but, used in combination with a board, enable clients to get further into the water. Clients with rheumatoid disease find frequently that lowering from the board to the seat requires more strength than they have in their upper limbs.

The fabric of the bath is important when considering the type of seat as fibreglass baths cannot cope with pressure from the seat being placed on their sides and there is a possibility that they may crack. Seats with supports that hang on the top of the bath are recommended for use in plastic baths.

The use of board and seat, while assisting clients to get over the bath, does have limitations caused primarily by the strength required to use them and the amount of strain placed through upper limbs. They do not get the client right down into the water, only allowing them to perch just above or just get below the level of the water. Some clients undoubtedly gain relief from pain and stiffness by soaking in warm water and this cannot be achieved by the use of board and seat.

Mechanical bath aids A range of mechanical bath aids exist which provide assistance for either the client or their carer. Some of these devices are static and others are portable and the mechanisms vary from springs to electricity. Several bath aids function on a spring basis, where the equipment is set according to the client's weight. The client transfers onto the seat and unlocks the mechanism which lowers into the bath. When the client has finished bathing a slight push on the side of the bath causes the mechanism to lift the client up out of the bath aided by the buoyancy of the water. Some of the mechanisms are more easy to use than others and controls placed more appropriately for clients with limited hand function. An aid like the Bathability is small and compact and can be easily transported if the client goes away from home.

Power-assisted bath aids utilize either electricity or power supplied by a rechargeable battery pack placed in the back rest. Either air or water is used to inflate a bellow located under the seat which raises the seat out of the bath level with the top enabling the client to transfer. The seat is deflated to lower the client into the bath. The control to operate the seat is relatively easy to use. Such equipment is usually portable and can be removed from the bath enabling other family members to bath unobstructed.

The main limitations of power-assisted aids are that they are quite heavy to lift and a carer who is elderly or has a disability may experience difficulty in removing them from the bath. They also have a solid back so that, while taking a client down further into the bath than a board and seat, they still do not enable the client to lie back in the water. These pieces of equipment may not be suitable for use in baths with anti-slip bottoms as the suction pads may not adhere to the bottom of the bath making them unstable to use.

Hand-wound mechanisms are also used to transfer clients into the bath. These comprise a seat which is raised and lowered and pivots around a central pole. The height to which the seat can be wound does vary and can have implications for clients with fixed flexion deformities of the knees. These clients need a seat which gives a greater clearance over the bath as they are unable to extend their knees to clear the bath.

Such equipment is more frequently used to assist carers as a lot of upper limb strength and movement is required to use it alone. Some of the seats also detach from the central pole fixing onto a chassis providing a portable chair as well. These are useful with clients who need more assistance to transfer or find being moved painful. The mobile chair can be wheeled to the bedside and the client transferred onto it. It has a commode aperture and is high enough to use over a toilet after which it can then be attached to the bath hoist the client transferred in and out of the bath and then used as a mobile chair again to wheel back into the bedroom. This avoids several transfers and fulfils the two functions of mobile commode chair and bath hoist.

Some of the winding mechanisms vary in their positioning making them more accessible for clients to use if they have limited upper limb strength, and some are powered by electricity which enables the client to raise the seat and traverse across the bath unaided.

Gel cushions are available, either to place on the bottom of the bath or on the seat of bath hoists to provide cushioning for clients with sacral nodules or pressure sores.

Overhead and mobile hoists   Clients who are more severely disabled may not be able to give any assistance in transferring and consideration should be given to either overhead or mobile hoists, used in combination with slings, to assist the carer. The use of mobile hoists can sometimes be limited in a bathroom due to a lack of space. To enable a mobile hoist to be positioned a section usually has to be removed from the bottom of the side panel of the bath so that the hoist can be pushed underneath. Mobile hoists do have the advantage of portability to assist with all transfers.

Slings are supportive and the hoists can lift up to an average of twenty stone with little effort on the carer's behalf. In a ward situation or in a client's home where all transfers are a problem a mobile hoist is more flexible as it can be used to assist with all transfers, whereas a ceiling-mounted hoist can only be used in the position in which it has been fixed. The design of quickfit slings requires very little movement of the client to position the sling and they can be positioned while the client is seated in a chair, whereas the more supportive hammock slings need to be positioned while the client is lying on a bed. There are a range of slings to use in combination with hoists, some canvas and some netting.

With much of the above equipment, except the winding mechanisms and hoists, the client when seated has to lift their legs over the bath and pivot round. If a client cannot do this easily, thought should be given to the stretch being applied to the skin on the client's bottom if twisted round by a carer. Torque and shear can easily cause a tear in fragile skin which may then develop into a pressure sore.

Showers   Showers will be discussed in relation to housing adaptations.

Personal hygiene

The main problems in relation to personal hygiene are:

- limited movement;
- weakness of grip;
- lack of dexterity.

Virtually all aspects of personal hygiene can be affected by rheumatoid disease. These activities are usually carried out either first thing in the morning, when joints can be stiff, or last thing at night, when pain and fatigue can limit function and are therefore highlighted frequently as problems areas. As they also involve aspects of personal care they may be highlighted as priorities as a means of maintaining dignity and are seen frequently as a high priority for the client.

Limited grip and dexterity
- razor handles can be padded or electric razors used;
- toothbrush handles can be padded with rubberzote or electric toothbrushes used;
- toothpaste dispensers can be wall mounted and require less pressure than squeezing the tube;
- showergel or liquid soap or soap on a rope overcomes handling slippery soap;
- stirex scissors assist with cutting nails;
- lever taps or tap turners enable taps to be turned on and off easily;
- sponges are more easily wrung out than flannels.

Limited upperlimb movement
- brushes, combs and other accessories can be purchased with extended handles;
- loofas can assist with washing backs;
- towelling bath robes help to dry the areas which cannot be reached;
- sheepskin washing brushes help to reach feet.

Toilets

The main problems in relation to toiletting are:

- transferring;
- cleansing after using the toilet;
- flushing the toilet;
- coping with clothing;
- use of sanitary protection;
- mobility to and from the toilet;
- use of public toilets.

131

Considerations

Independence in toiletting is a priority for many clients as assistance can be embarrassing and demeaning. For clients who are experiencing minimal difficulty in toiletting the range of equipment available can often overcome problems and regain independence. It is when a client is having difficulty in getting to or transferring from the toilet that problems become more complex to solve. In this situation the amount of assistance available is of primary importance and will influence the solution arrived at. The problems created by dependence in toiletting can be immense especially for clients living alone as highlighted by the following case.

A lady with severe rheumatoid disease was admitted to hospital and underwent a below knee amputation due to vasculitis and impaired circulation. She was unable to use a prosthesis as she had neither the upper or lower limb function to do so and the weakness of her upper limbs made transferring independently impossible. She was provided with an electric wheelchair and regained some mobility. She lived alone and a home assessment was carried out. All aspects of her care could be covered apart from toiletting. Nurses called to get her up in the morning, home helps and meals on wheels called during the day and nurses called to put her to bed at night. This was at a time when home helps were unable to provide assistance with personal care, and this situation has now changed in this lady's locality.

The two remaining problems were: what happened from 10.00am–7.00pm between visits from the nurse and also what happened during the evening and night, in respect to using the toilet? One solution was to provide an electric wheelchair with an integral commode, but this presented problems with sacral pressure care, the client felt it totally unacceptable, not only in terms of the necessary clothing adaptations but also in terms of dignity and hygiene. She did not have the manual dexterity to use a female urinal. The day time was eventually overcome by a rota of carers from friends and the voluntary sector calling throughout the day.

The evening still remained however. The client tried numerous female urinals and positions and eventually a custom made device was produced which she could use with a great deal of effort. Her daughter also decided to travel every night to help toilet her before she went to sleep. The discharge from hospital was very tenuous and the main reason was trying to cope with a client's personal care needs with a limited resource. The option which had been considered at one point was residential care purely through a client's inability to toilet independently.

Transfers

If a client is mobile but is having difficulty getting on and off of the toilet a raised toilet seat can provide the extra height needed to reduce stress on joints. The height on the seat can vary from two to six inches and the seats should be secured to avoid slipping when in use. Front cutouts enable clients with limited arm movement to cleanse themselves from the front instead of behind. A seat can be obtained with either the front left or right side shaped to accommodate a client who has a fixed hip and is unable to flex it to 90°. If the extra height is not enough to assist a client to stand, a self-lift toilet seat can be used which provides a spring seat which, as with self-lift chairs, is set according to the client's weight.

If stability is needed grab rails fitted beside the toilet will provide more assistance. If the wall is not strong enough to fix rails to a free-standing or preferably a floor fixed frame can provide an armrest on either side of the client to assist with transfers. Frames which combine a seat as well as armgrips can be used. These are usually adjustable in height and can be either free-standing or floor fixed. If the frame is free-standing the client must be taught to use both arm-rests when transferring to avoid the frame tipping.

If a client has limited mobility and is using a wheelchair enough space must be available to enable the chair to be positioned correctly for the client to transfer or for carers to assist without being cramped. It is possible for some clients to maintain their independence with the use of an overhead tracking hoist in combination with a sling with a commode aperture.

Some clients are unable to transfer and are totally reliant upon outside agencies for their assistance. In this situation an alternative means of toiletting is needed as bladder and bowel function cannot be totally dependent upon the visit of the care attendant. Several options exist, probably the most desirable is the use of a U-shaped cushion in the wheelchair which allows for a urinal to be inserted and used while sitting in the wheelchair. The success of this method is dependent upon the client's manual dexterity to position the urinal and remove it, adapted clothing is also required to overcome problems of pants and tights.

Wheelchairs which combine commodes are available but do have some limitations. Some clients, understandably, find the use of wheelchair commodes embarrassing as talking to a visitor while seated on a commode which you have just used can be distressing. The other problem which these pose is that of pressure. Although the seats are padded, areas of high pressure can be caused around the rim of the aperture. In some situations however the use of a wheelchair commode can be the difference between remaining at home or needing residential or long-term hospital care.

Cleansing after using the toilet

Limitation in upper limb movement, manual dexterity or external rotation of the hip can all be causes of problems in cleansing after using the toilet. Upper limb movement can be compensated for by the use of long handled toilet paper holders which can be used from the front. Tearing off toilet paper can be overcome by using toilet tissues rather than roll. Limited movement of the hips can be more of a problem and may require the use of a bidet. A Clos O Mat toilet provides the facilities for a person with severe limitations of movement to operate a warm water douche to cleanse themselves and then use warm air to dry themselves.

Flushing toilets

Sometimes clients can experience difficulty in operating toilet flushes and adaptations are needed to either bring chains within reach or provide a different grip.

Coping with clothes

Adjusting clothes can be a problem for some clients. Zips and buttons on trousers may need to be adapted. A small piece of tape or a safety pin threaded through the eye of a zip enables a better grip upon the pull. Velcro fastening to replace buttons may also be needed. If women have problems in pulling tights up and down, stockings or stay-ups eliminate the need to remove them while using the toilet. French knickers are more easy to pull up and down than tight cotton pants.

Coping with sanitary protection

The use of sanitary protection may become difficult if hands are painful and grip or upper limb movement limited. Tampons with an applicator may be more easy to use. If this is difficult then sanitary towels with self adhesive backings may be more convenient.

Mobility to and from the toilet

Limitation in mobility can lead to the need for alternative toiletting arrangements to be considered. Some clients experience limited mobility during the night when they are perhaps feeling stiff and moving more slowly. In this situation a bedside commode may be appropriate. Some clients may be completely unable to gain access to the bathroom, perhaps because they can no longer get upstairs, and need a more permanent arrangement. While commodes may be provided initially their acceptability will depend upon the availability of people to empty them. Chemical toilets provide a more acceptable alternative as they can be flushed after use and require less frequent emptying than commodes, lasting several days. They can be set upon platforms to provide height and armrests and some are now produced in the form of a chair with padded back support and a wood finish. The use of mobile chairs enable carers to get clients to the bathroom more quickly and some are high enough to be wheeled over the toilet decreasing the need to transfer.

Using public toilets

The difficulty in using public toilets or in reaching the toilet in a friend's house can deter people from going out for any length of time or lead them to limit their fluid intake. While more buildings are now offering adapted toilets many clients still worry about finding an accessible toilet. Small hand-held urinals, or bottles for men can overcome the problem of accessibility or being unable to rise from a low toilet. Problems have also been experienced in relation to the heavy locks and doors which public buildings frequently install and clients have relayed examples of being locked in toilets and having to call for assistance to get out. While these situations can often be looked back upon and laughed at they are a cause of stress and embarrassment and may deter clients from going out in the future.

Beds

The main problems in relation to beds are:

- transfers;
- comfort;
- pressure relief.

Considerations

If a client is experiencing difficulties in relation to any of the above it is likely that they and their partners are experiencing regular sleep disturbance. This can range from being woken once every so many nights to being awoken several times each night. The level of fatigue experienced from loss of sleep can have a profound effect on both client and carer. The awareness, on the client's behalf, of disturbing their partner's sleep can lead to the decision to sleep in separate beds or different rooms.

This isolation can be even greater for the client who is unable to cope with stairs and has to move a bed downstairs while their partner sleeps upstairs. Isolation caused by lack of sleep can be experienced when a client, who is not sleeping during the night, sleeps for long periods through the day to catch up, thus sleeping while the family is awake and being awake when the family is asleep.

If a client is spending a lot of time in bed a special bed may be needed to enable the client to adjust their position independently, assist carers with transfers or care functions and provide pressure relief. It is difficult to assist with many care functions in a double bed which is not adjustable in position or height and where easy access to both sides of the bed may not be possible.

Transfers The main problem of getting into bed is often raising legs up onto the mattress and the problem with getting out is rising from a low base. Small spiral steps called bedhoppers are available to enable clients to work their legs up onto the bed in stages. The height of beds can be increased by the use of blocks or raises. However raising the height may assist with getting up but make getting in more difficult.

Comfort and pressure relief Comfort can be affected by pain, stiffness and the presence of nodules. Muscle wasting and loss of weight can also add to pressure problems.

Clients often buy orthopaedic mattresses but these do not necessarily provide the right amount of support. A firm hard mattress does not accommodate the curves of the body and areas of high pressure can be caused at contact points. A soft spongey mattress on the other hand provides no support and the body is enveloped in it making transfers difficult and providing little support. A guide to the required amount of support is to lie flat on the back and try to slip an arm under the lumbar curve. If it slides through easily the mattress is too firm, if the pelvis has to be arched to get it through the mattress is too soft. The arm should slide through with a small amount of movement required.

Bed paddings are an effective way of providing cushioning for painful joints. They are placed on top of the mattress and are usually made of fibre filling. They can be purchased with a plastic or material covering. If this padding is to be used at home it may be worth considering the use of a segmented mattress as these are more easily laundered. The sections can be removed from the cover and the cover washed like a sheet. Sheepskin fleeces also provide a degree of comfort for painful joints.

Special pressure-relieving mattresses can be obtained for clients who are at high risk of developing pressure sores. These can be air filled, or floatation and provide a higher degree of pressure relief than ordinary mattresses or fleeces.

CLOTHING

The main problems are in relation to limited movement and poor dexterity. Limited shoulder movement can present difficulties with back fastenings, such as bras and zips on dresses, getting arms into jumpers, shirts and blouses and reaching to dress lower limbs. Poor dexterity can present problems in relation to fastenings. Limited lower limb movement can lead to difficulties in dressing the lower half of the body.

Front fastening clothes are usually easier to cope with as are clothes which are not a tight fit. The weight of clothes is also a consideration, especially when buying such garments as winter coats. Elasticated girdles or support stockings present problems as they require a strong grip to pull on and even to use in conjunction with dressing aids. Helping hands and dressing sticks can provide extra reach and assist in removing clothes from shoulders or pulling clothes onto the shoulders.

One client related how she was having difficulty in getting her winter coat onto her shoulders and so hung it over the knob at the bottom of the staircase so that she could just slip her arms into it and shrug it onto her shoulders. Having placed her arms into it she was unable to get it onto her shoulders and was left attached to the bannister until someone came to release her; she welcomed the idea of a dressing stick!

Stocking gutters can assist with stockings, tights or socks, although for some clients the finger dexterity required to use these may be too great. Button hooks can assist with doing up buttons, or velcro fastening can be used to replace the button completely.

Long handled shoe horns and elastic laces may assist clients who are having difficulties getting their shoes on and off. Involvement of the metatarsal joints can lead to pain and difficulty in walking. Insoles which have been specially moulded to the client's feet may provide some padding or be built-up in such a way as to redistribute the points of pressure and weight bearing when walking. These insert into shoes which can cause problems for some clients. The shoe may not be designed to take the extra thickness of an insert and this will lead to increased pressure on the top of the toes as they are being pushed upwards. It may be necessary to buy new shoes which accommodate the insert.

Cushioned sole and arch support is provided by many makes of trainers and the softness of the uppershoe accommodates deformity. Some clients feel happier wearing trainers than specially made orthopaedic shoes which can be limited in their design. However some clients will need to have orthopaedic shoes made to accommodate deformities which may have developed and limit the range of shop made shoes available to them. Extra ankle support may be needed to prevent inversion from occurring or arch support needed.

MOBILITY

Problems in relation to mobility can be experienced due to limited movement, pain and stiffness, fatigue and contractures of the lower limbs. The choice of footwear has already been discussed, the use of walking aids, the need to use manual or electric wheelchairs to increase mobility or the adaptation of a car to make driving more easy will now be considered.

Walking aids

The use of some walking aids can be made difficult by the grip required to hold them, the strain placed upon joints while using them or the strength needed to move them. Specially moulded handles are available for sticks and crutches which distribute the pressure more evenly over the whole hand.

A frequent request regards the suitability of sticks which open out into a seat. Several different models are on the market, some more stable than others when used as a seat. Clients feel it advantageous to have their own seat with them if they require a rest, but the stability of the seat should be ascertained.

The use of elbow crutches or walking sticks can cause pain in the wrist and elbows as pressure is exerted through them. This can be reduced by the use of gutter crutches and pulpit frames which provide support along the length of the forearm, through which the weight is borne. If a client finds lifting walking frames difficult casters enable the frame to be glided rather than lifted.

If a client uses a frame to walk with the ability to fold the frame may be advantageous. When travelling in cars, frames can take up a lot of space and limit the number of passengers. Folding frames collapse flat and can be stored in the boot allowing more room in the car.

Various types of rollators and walking frames are available which incorporate a seat to rest on when tired or a tray to assist with carrying items around.

Manual wheelchairs

When a client's mobility becomes impaired to the extent that it is limiting their ability to go out they may decide to use a wheelchair to enhance their mobility over long distances. A range of self-propelling and attendant controlled chairs are available through the District Health Authority and is supplied free of cost to the client.

The range of lightweight chairs is extending rapidly and some clients do choose to purchase their own chair for several reasons. The prime reason is often the ease of manœuvrability of the chair. The centre of gravity of the chair can usually be altered to enable the chair to be tipped more easily for mounting kerbs. If the wheelchair user has the upper limb strength to balance on the back wheels of the chair they can mount kerbs unassisted and gain a greater degree of independence. Even if the client is unable to do this, propelling the chair is much easier. Most wheelchair manufacturers are now producing lightweight wheelchairs which are easy to propel and manœuvre and light to lift in and out of a car. They often dismantle into small components, the wheels being quick release, which means that they take up less storage space.

The main disadvantage of private purchase is that the maintenance and replacement of the chair is the client's responsibility as is the supply of any special cushion which they may require. Chairs supplied by the DSA are maintained, replaced and special seating needs assessed at no cost to the client. A secondary consideration for some clients is also the design and colour range which is available through private purchase.

Powered wheelchairs

The strength needed to self-propel is substantial and some clients may be unable to use a manual wheelchair for this reason. Powered mobility offers clients a greater degree of independence in this situation. Sometimes a client's carer may not have the strength to push a chair and for this reason seek the assistance of power.

The range of chairs available starts with an indoor powered chair, which is purely for use inside, then moves on to an indoor/outdoor chair, which is compact and manœuvrable enough to use in a house but also has the facility to cope with kerbs and outdoor environments, and finally finishes with an outdoor chair which is usually more powerful and robust, can cope with longer journeys, but does not provide the manœuvrability in confined environments.

Indoor chairs are supplied through the wheelchair services after an assessment has been carried out. However, at the moment they do not supply an outdoor electric wheelchair which can be used independently or offer the facility to cope with kerbs and travel long distances. This situation is under review. They do supply an attendant controlled chair which is large and cumbersome and does not reflect the vast improvements in technology over recent years.

For some clients the cost of powered chairs is prohibitive, especially if the client is not eligible for or in receipt of a mobility allowance. It is sometimes possible to seek assistance with funding from charitable trusts and organizations who frequently contribute to the cost of such equipment. However if funding is sought in this way consideration must be given to the cost of maintaining, insuring and replacing the chair once purchased.

A wide range of powered chairs are on the market and clients should try several before deciding upon the final purchase. Disabled Living Centres usually keep a range of chairs for demonstration, the range will depend upon the size of the centre, but all will have a wide variety of manufacturer's literature. It is essential that clients have a home demonstration of the chair before they make a final purchase to ensure that the chair is appropriate for the environment in which it is going to be used. The addition of kerb climbers can increase the overall width of the chair making manœuvrability more difficult, access to and from the home must be assessed and access to points to recharge the battery considered.

The chairs are powered by a rechargeable battery which is charged using mains electricity. The range of the chair will vary from chair to chair and it is worth remembering that the range quoted on the literature often refers to the distance the chair will travel on the flat. Coping with hilly environments will decrease this overall distance.

The controls for the chairs are usually simple to operate comprising an on/off switch, a joystick for steering and a speed control. A sustained grip is required to keep the chair moving and for some clients this can be a problem if they are travelling several miles. The controls can be located on either the left or right hand side, some are multi-adjustable in height and distance from the end of the arm, while others are positioned on purchase and relocation requires work from the supplier. Clients with limited movement, grip or hand function may need the controls positioned in a different place from the arm rest to enable ease of access.

The ability to climb kerbs provides clients with a much greater degree of independence, as not all pavements are dropped to allow ease of crossing. Kerb climbers are situated in several different positions: on the front wheels, on the outside of the front wheels, in the middle of the foot rest. Some chairs do not require kerb climbers. Kerb climbers can add extra width to the chairs and for this reason some manufacturers offer the option of indoor and outdoor footrests, one with and one without kerb climbers. Kerb climbers situated in the middle of the footrest, while reducing the overall width of the chair, can impair transfers, depending on how the client transfers. Some chairs are front wheel drive and usually have large front wheels which have the power to climb kerbs. It is necessary to consider the implications for clients who have cervical involvement and wish to use an outdoor chair as the process of kerb climbing can jar the neck and may have contra-indications depending upon the degree of cervical instability.

One of the problems associated with powered chairs is their portability. Many chairs do dismantle to fit into a car but, even when dismantled, the components are extremely heavy. This can be prohibitive to some clients whose carers cannot cope with lifting.

More and more clients are opting to buy scooters rather than powered chairs. They have the ability to travel similar distances and to cope with kerbs and, like chairs, differ in their suitability for different environments. They are also powered by batteries. Again a sustained grip is needed to operate the scooter and there is a larger degree of variability between models in the grip required. The size of scooters can prohibit access to some buildings. Clients who have some degree of mobility use scooters to travel long distances to and from shops being able to walk around the shop once they arrive. Scooters are perceived as being more socially acceptable than wheelchairs and also have the bonus of being less expensive.

The other form of powered mobility available are buggy type vehicles. These vehicles are large and purely for outdoor use requiring garaging and access to power to recharge batteries. These vehicles do give a much greater degree of weather protection and again are more suitable for clients who have a degree of mobility as access to buildings is a major problem.

Clients buying some form of powered vehicle should be encouraged to take out an insurance policy including third party cover, as it is possible that they could be involved in an accident.

Car adaptations

Limitations in movement, grip strength or dexterity can all lead to problems with driving. The ability to drive offers a great degree of independence and clients who are already in possession of a licence can carry out adaptations to maintain their independence in most situations. The onus is placed upon the client to inform the DVLC at Swansea of any disability which they have, although some clients are reluctant to do this for fear of losing their licence.

Some of the main problems experienced by clients relate to limited foot movement, poor grip due to swan neck or other deformities of the hand, limited neck movement due to cervical involvement and access to and from the car.

Automatic transmission overcomes many of the problems associated with pedal control and also limits the amount of upperlimb movement needed in relation to gear changes. Poor grip can lead to problems in gripping the steering wheel which may be overcome by the use of a pommel or knob being attached onto the wheel. Weakness of grip can cause problems with using the hand break which can be adapted or repositioned. Limitations in neck movement can be compensated for by the use of extra mirrors in the car providing all round visibility. Access to and from the car can be difficult for clients with severely limited movement, especially if they require assistance with transfers. Existing car seats can be replaced by swivel car seats which rotate round out of the car to enable a client to do a side transfer from a wheelchair or for carers to assist more easily with transfer. Once the client has transferred onto the seat it is rotated back around into the car. Limitation in upper limb movement may also present difficulties in relation to using a seat belt. Adaptations can be made to belts to bring them into the reach of a person with limited shoulder movement.

One of the problems experienced by non-drivers is identifying driving instructors who have adapted cars on which to learn. Local instructors with limited adaptations are usually identifiable. Clients with a greater degree of disability may require a specific assessment of their limitations and abilities to establish exactly what adaptations are required to assist them to drive and these are carried out at assessment centres such as Banstead Place Mobility Centre.

Home management

Assistive devices to help with aspects of home management are as numerous as the problems encountered by clients in relation to this aspect of function. This section will provide a broad perspective of both and not an exhaustive list. Comparisons of some categories of equipment have been documented in DHSS equipment reports and are available on request.

Opening bottles and jars

Opening bottles, jars and cans is an area of difficulty experienced by many clients. Jars and bottle openers are either hand held or wall mounted. Hand held devices range from a non-slip pad to plier like devices. The amount of grip required to operate these devices varies and in some cases is prohibitive. Wall mounted versions can be V-shaped to grip the top of varying size jars or bell shaped with non-slip rubber inside. The positioning of these devices is important to allow for maximum pressure to be applied. Rubber grips can also be purchased which fit onto individual bottle tops to enlarge the grip required to open them.

Opening cans

For many clients electric can-openers are the most effective way of opening cans, requiring little grip or hand strength. Many have a lever action and if the lever is large then the heel of the hand or the forearm can be used to operate.

Plugs

Pulling electric plugs in and out of the socket or reaching the socket can cause problems. Plugs can be purchased with large handles on them to enable the whole hand to be used, rather than just the finger tips. Extension brackets can be plugged into sockets near the floor and wall mounted to bring the socket within the reach of clients with restricted movement.

Taps

Lever action taps are easier to use as they place less stress on the fingers. Tap turners can be used to adapt existing taps if replacement is too costly, they can be fitted to ordinary or crystal taps. If clients are replacing taps with lever mechanisms, ones which have 180° turn provide more control over the volume of water coming out of the tap than the 90° mechanism.

Saucepans

Problems related to lifting saucepans can be overcome by placing vegetables etc. in cooking baskets, so that when they are cooked they can be lifted from the pan negating the need to carry pan and water and also to drain them. The use of microwaves can reduce significantly the amount of lifting of heavy hot utensils in the kitchen.

Kettles

Filling can be made easier by using a plastic jug, rather than carrying a heavy full kettle. Problems associated with lifting and pouring can be overcome by, using a kettle tipper, tippers are now available for jug as well as conventional kettles using a smaller travelling kettle or a microwave to make drinks in. Small drinks dispensers are also available from large department stores.

Utensils

The handles of utensils can be padded for clients with restricted grip, or ranges of knives are available with the handles in different positions placing less strain on the wrist when in use. The grip of utensils should be considered when buying equipment as often conventional ranges can offer a better grip, rather than having to buy specific equipment designed for people with disabilities.

Cooker and heating controls

A range of adaptations for controls are available for appliances. The Gas and Electricity Boards provide a range of alternative controls for appliances. Individual grips can be moulded by the use of a Grip Kit which enables a handle to be moulded in a maluable material which then sets forming a rigid grip.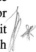

The range of equipment to assist in home management tasks is immense. It is not the intention of this chapter to list every item available but to provide an indication of the range and of considerations that should be taken into account. Proper assessment for assistive equipment is essential to ensure that appropriate equipment is provided that will meet the physical, psychological, social and environmental needs of the client and their family. Ideally this should take place in the client's home although it is appreciated that this is not always possible.

As the commercial market for equipment is growing, client's awareness of equipment is being raised through advertising in the popular press. This has both advantages and disadvantages. The advantages are that clients are now beginning to take initiatives in requesting help because they are now aware that help does exist, they are more informed about the choice that they have and they can place pressure on local authorities to provide more than a basic range of equipment. Clients are now beginning to ask 'why is that not available through Social Services?' The answer is often difficult to explain.

The biggest disadvantage, however, is that the scope for parting with large amounts of money for inappropriate equipment has also become larger. Clients may not be prepared to wait for a therapist assessment or may prefer to purchase privately and many clients are being encountered who have purchased expensive items of equipment following a demonstration from a company representative and found the equipment to be unsuitable. The increase in commercial centres

145

and high street shops selling equipment widens the potential for errors to be made, however many of the new retail outlets either employ therapists or use therapists to train staff and are aware of the potential to not only waste a client's money but also in some cases cause harm.

Assessment should ensure that appropriate equipment is provided and kept to a minimum. A factor which is often neglected due to lack of therapist time is that needs change and equipment may either no longer be needed or may need reassessing. This is often left to the client to report and the assumption made that if the client has not been in contact the equipment must be alright. While a routine reassessment is out of the question therapists should ensure that clients know who to contact if their needs change or if the equipment breaks down.

FURTHER READING

M. Brattstrom (1987) *Joint Protection and Rehabilitation in Chronic Rheumatic Disorders*, Wolfe Medical Publications Ltd, London.

J. Melvin (1977) *Rheumatic Diseases: Occupational Therapy and Rehabilitation*, F.A. Davis Company.

H. Unsworth (1986) *Coping with Rheumatoid Arthritis*, Chambers.

7

Housing adaptation

The need to consider housing adaptation becomes apparent when the physical environment in which the client functions becomes a barrier to maintaining previous levels of function for the client or when a combination of the client's condition and the environment inhibit the functioning of a carer or the family unit and these situations cannot be met by the provision of assistive equipment. Clients may not wish to be rehoused, if in local authority accommodation, or to move house for a variety of reasons, apart from the upheaval involved. If the client has a young family, moving will invariably affect children's schooling that may necessitate them moving to a different school. If the client has lived in an area for a long period of time support and friendships may exist within the local community which would be lost if the client moved house. This factor becomes even more important if the client is elderly, a situation which is frequently encountered in an elderly population is a client being rehoused and slowly losing contact with their friends and the local community as mobility becomes a problem for all concerned. The extent of a housing adaptation can vary from the installation of a walk in shower in a bathroom to building a downstairs extension containing bedroom and bathroom facilities.

Communication and co-operation between therapist, client, housing department, environmental health inspector and architect, if appropriate, is essential to ensure that the appropriate adaptation is carried out and the process of application for grants, funding and planning permission is as smooth as possible. Adaptations should be carried out with longterm prognosis in mind. While it is difficult to predict outcome in relation to rheumatoid disease its progressive nature should be borne in mind, as far as possible, to prevent the need for costly revision of adaptations if the client's condition changes. The policies and procedures for carrying out housing adaptations varies enormously from local authority to local authority and so it is not the intention of this section to consider in detail specific policies and procedures: therapists should familiarize themselves with local procedures relevant to their work.

Occupational therapists can be involved in adaptation to a variety of different properties including:

1. local authority housing;
2. privately rented accommodation;
3. owner occupied accommodation;
4. new local authority housing schemes.

The whole process of grant applications, architect's visits and fees, responsibilities regarding redecorating or installing extra central heating can be a minefield of confusion for clients. It is essential that therapists spend time with the family to explain the procedures involved, the costs which the client will be expected to contribute to, any implications for increased bills in the future as in heating an extension, and the length of time the whole process will take. Clients should also be informed of the amount of upheaval that will occur during building or installation so that the necessary plans can be made during that time.

Assessment and identification of need

Assessment and identification of need is a responsibility of all local authorities. This responsibility is laid down in the Chronically Sick and Disabled Persons Act 1970. Section 1 of the Chronically Sick and Disabled Persons Act requires authorities to inform themselves of the number of people with disabilities in their area and of their need for services, to publish information about available services and inform users of other services which may be of relevance to them. The act then goes on to identify specific services which include transport, recreation, meals and practical assistance in the home. In relation to housing adaptation and equipment it states that local authorities must make arrangements for:

the provision of assistance for that person in arranging for the carrying out of any works of adaptation in his home or the provision of any additional facilities designed to secure his greater safety, comfort or convenience.

The way in which this act is interpreted varies considerably from authority to authority. Obviously authorities are working with financial constraints and budgets have to be allocated accordingly. Conflict arises when the needs perceived by the therapist and client differ in their perception of importance or when the needs identified by the therapist conflict with the existing policy of the employing authority. A clear assessment procedure is needed to ensure that specific aims and objectives are identified and prioritized. Communication is vitally important to ensure that the client knows exactly what is being proposed, what is entailed and why the specific decisions have been reached. This factor becomes more important in the light of the Disabled Persons (Services, Consultation and Representation) Act 1986 which in section 1 identifies the provision of a procedure to appoint a representative for a person with a disability and establishes guidelines for the rights of that representative stating that if required an authority must supply a written statement, 'either specifying:

(a) (i) any needs of the disabled person which in the opinion of the authority call for the provision by them of any statutory services and;
   (ii) in the case of each such need, the statutory services that they propose to provide to meet the need;
      or stating that, in their opinion, the disabled person has no needs calling for the provision by them of any such services and;
(b) giving an explanation of their decision'

While not all of the sections of this act have as yet been implemented it will provide clients with a procedure of appeal and representation and make local authorities and therapists more accountable for their decisions and actions. This act also states that in all assessments for the provision of services to disabled people the needs of carers must also be taken into account. This section will now go on to look at specific adaptations which may be needed for a client with rheumatoid disease.

KITCHEN DESIGN AND ADAPTATION

The need to adapt a kitchen for clients with rheumatoid disease is often encountered if a client has made the transition from being ambulant to using a wheelchair and therefore the layout of the kitchen needs adapting to compensate for the client's new position of function. In some situations a client may have the opportunity to re-design their kitchen, when redecorating or moving home, and may be seeking advice on factors which need to be considered to make kitchen activities easier to cope with.

The factors which need to be considered are the needs and abilities of the client, the use of the kitchen, the needs of other people who may be using the kitchen, design considerations and the existing physical environment of the kitchen. While publications provide anthropometric data it should be remembered that these data are guidelines and a therapist involved in a kitchen adaptation for an individual client has the opportunity to tailor make a kitchen to the needs of the individual.

The needs and abilities of the client are fundamental to kitchen design. This means establishing the functional abilities and disabilities of the client and what they feel to be important factors to consider. Functions which may be limited for a client with rheumatoid disease are discussed below.

Reach

The ability to reach into wall cupboards and lift something down may be limited as may the ability to reach across work surfaces by decreased range of movement in the upper limbs, or decreased strength. If a person is in a wheelchair their ability to reach will be compromised not only by possible upper limb involvement but also by the fact that they are functioning from a seated position.

Ability to bend

Poor balance and limited hip movement may make bending down to cupboards, plug sockets, or the bottom of the fridge, cooker or other appliance difficult. Knee movement and pain may mean that clients can no longer kneel on the floor. This will also be the case if a client has undergone a total knee arthroplasty.

Stamina

Levels of fatigue may make standing for any period of time difficult and many kitchen activities may need to be carried out sitting down. Muscle weakness may make standing for prolonged periods difficult.

Hand function

This may limit the client's ability to use controls, switches plugs, taps, open cupboards, etc.

Mobility

If the client is using an aid to mobility this may affect the amount of circulation space needed in the kitchen.

Other factors which need to be considered are how much the client is intending to use the kitchen and what for. The level of use will range from needing to make a drink or a snack to needing to prepare all the family meals and carry out other domestic activities such as laundry. The possible longterm prognosis of rheumatoid disease is also a consideration. If the kitchen is being planned for an ambulant person it may be worth using a kitchen unit which allows for easy repositioning of height should the client at some point need to use a wheelchair. The flexibility of units heights is an important factor if considering a kitchen which will be used by different occupants as in local authority housing schemes. Repositioning enables the same kitchen to be used whether the client is ambulant or uses a wheelchair. Although the initial cost may be more the flexibility negates the need to refurbish the kitchen to meet the needs of a new tenant.

The use to which the kitchen is put is also another factor to consider. For many people the kitchen fulfils a much greater role than that of a food preparation area. It may also be a dining area, or the focal point of the home in which friends are entertained, children play and television is watched. Many kitchens also provide access to the garden, utility room or garage; all of these factors can influence ultimate design.

In a family situation usually more than one person uses the kitchen area and the needs of other family members are important. In some situations decisions have to be taken as to who the kitchen is being designed for. For example a client who is using a wheelchair will have very different design needs to that of her mobile husband and adolescent children. Is the kitchen to be designed totally around the needs of the client or will some compromises be made to accommodate the needs of his or her family? In a group home situation the kitchen area may be used by several people all with different disabilities and needs and some compromises may be needed.

Design considerations relate firstly to whether the identified needs can be met using the existing area of the kitchen, whether it will be necessary to utilize space from an adjacent room or whether there is an indication that an extension is needed and if the space is available for this option. Problems are encountered frequently in relation to clients who use a wheelchair in finding the space necessary for circulation.

Specific design considerations relate to storage units, work surfaces, sinks, switches and sockets, lighting, flooring and appliances.

Base storage units are needed to provide easy access to items on shelves and at the back of cupboards to overcome problems in bending or balance. This can be achieved in several ways, the shelves can be on runners so that they slide out making items more easy to see and avoiding having to bend down so far. The space often wasted by corner units can be utilized by the use of a carousel rather than shelving. This revolving shelf unit allows easy access to items on the shelf as well as utilizing what would otherwise have been wasted space. Locating storage baskets on the inside of cupboard doors can also provide accessible shelving. The hinges on base unit doors should be as strong as possible as many clients will use them to steady themselves with as they bend down. Some units are designed with this specifically in mind.

Access to wall cupboards frequently presents problems for clients with limited reach. While items can be organized so that the items used most frequently are placed on the lower shelves access to all shelving is rarely gained. This can be achieved by the use of units with shelving which can be pulled out of the cupboard and down within reach and then returned to the cupboard when finished with. Limited reach above the head is a common problem for clients with rheumatoid disease, as is having the upper limb strength to reach up and to hold a heavy object.

Clients who are working from a wheelchair lose access often to a great deal of storage space. Floor units are compromised to enable access to work surfaces, sinks or hobs and wall cupboards can become inaccessible due to their height. Mobile trolleys fitting under the work surface do provide some storage space to help overcome this problem. Units can be purchased with pull-out work surfaces so that a client in a wheelchair has access to an appropriate surface as well as maintaining the cupboard space of base units.

Most suppliers of kitchen units for people with disabilities offer a wide range of door handles and fittings usually offering different diameters and different shapes to enable a range of grips to be considered.

The heights of work surface will vary according to the position from which the client is working. In a family kitchen, if the client is a wheelchair user, it may be necessary to provide a range of heights to provide for the needs of other family members. As well as considering the height of the work surface it is also necessary to consider the clearance beneath the surface if the client is working from a wheelchair or seated position. There must be enough room for the chair to be drawn close to the unit or the arms of the chair to fit underneath, depending on how close the client needs to be to work. Alternatively consideration can be given to providing desk arms to the wheelchair enabling closer access to working surfaces. Clearance for the footplates of wheelchairs should be considered also. The depth of the unit is important for clients with limited reach as this may affect access to power points and utensils at the back of the surface.

Other factors which need to be considered are as follows.

1. The depth of the sink, especially if the client is working from a wheelchair.
2. The position of the draining board, clients usually have a preference to left or right.
3. The type of taps used, preferably lever for ease of operation.
4. The position of power points and whether they are accessible.
5. The use of both natural and artificial light.
6. The type of flooring to be used, whether it is non-slip.

The overall design of the kitchen should be considered not only in terms of functional ability but also in terms of work flow. This is especially important for people with rheumatoid disease ensuring that the relationship of appliances and storage units and sink reflect the principles of energy conservation minimizing the amount of energy being put into food preparation.

Appliances

It is not intended to go into specific consideration for all appliances used in a kitchen as this is well documented in other publications. Factors which need to be considered as a general guideline are:

1. overall position of the appliance in the kitchen to maximize work flow;
2. access to shelves in terms of height, especially ovens, fridges and freezers;
3. ease of use of appliance.

Overall position

Appliances should be positioned to minimize the amount of movement between them. Thought should be given to the proximity of work surfaces to minimize the distance items have to be carried. Specific surfaces may be located in close proximity to appliances like ovens. A pull-out work surface is often located under the oven in an oven-casing to provide a surface to rest hot dishes on.

Access to appliance

The height at which appliances are situated can determine how accessible they are. Placing fridges in built in units allows them to be situated above floor level giving easy access to all shelves. A split level cooker provides easy access to ovens, many clients find bending to lift dishes from the oven very difficult and dangerous. Upright deep freezes provide easier access to the contents than the chest type, as less bending and reach is required to use them.

Ease of use

The type of controls on appliances are an important consideration when purchasing as is the ease of cleaning.

The inclusion by *Which?* of a section relating to people with special needs in some of their consumer reports is a welcome addition. Clients will now have access to a comprehensive consumer report on a range of readily available products enabling them to identify specific points before purchasing a major appliance for the home. It is very difficult for some clients to do the rounds of showrooms to examine a range of products and assistants do not always know the answers to specific questions a client may have.

BATHROOM ADAPTATION

Problems in relation to personal hygiene can be overcome often by the use of assistive equipment which has already been discussed, however, adaptations are sometimes required. The most common forms of bathroom adaptation for clients with rheumatoid disease are the installation of showers or the relocation of the bathroom on the ground floor. The main problems encountered by clients are:

1. mobility
   - access to the bathroom during the day can be difficult if it is located upstairs;
   - Clients using aids to mobility may find their bathroom too small to manoeuvre the aid around in;
2. inability/difficulty to transfer due to pain, stiffness or loss of movement;
3. problems with cleansing after using the toilet.

As with kitchen design it is necessary to consider the needs of the family in planning a bathroom adaptation to ensure that all needs are taken into consideration. The installation of a shower in a small bathroom may mean that the bath is removed, inevitably effecting the whole family. Another important area to consider is the needs of the carer if assistance is needed with personal hygiene. Adequate space should be provided to assist with transfers and other aspects of care. If assistance with washing is needed a system should be provided that does not require the carer to put on waterproofs in order to assist!

Mobility

Access to and around the bathroom can pose problems. The provision of a stairlift is a common way of gaining access to the bathroom, if upstairs, during the day. However in some homes the stairs may not be suitable for the installation of a lift and the provision of a downstairs bathroom and bedroom may be considered.

The use of walking frames and wheelchairs in bathrooms can be

155

inhibited by the size of some rooms, especially if the bath and toilet are in separate rooms. It is necessary sometimes to remove dividing walls to gain a greater circulation space, if the problem cannot be overcome by the provision of more compact aids to mobility, and to provide adequate space for transfer to be carried out safely.

Transfers

Bathing

The provision of assistive equipment to assist with transfers in the bath has already been discussed, for some clients however the provision of a shower may be preferable. Even with assistive equipment clients may need assistance to swing their legs up over the side of the bath and still be dependent upon assistance from a carer. Many bath aids have rigid backs preventing the upper body from being immersed in the warm water. Some clients prefer the overall warmth provided by a shower as they feel it relieves pain and stiffness.

A large variety of shower trays exist which provide level access to the shower, either to walk in to or to use in combination with a mobile shower chair. The main consideration in relation to the size of the tray is whether the client is ambulant or a wheelchair user. The type of shower installed varies considerably from a non-slip tiled floor with a central drain to a shower cubicle depending on the constraints of the client's bathroom and the policy of the local authority. Some of the showers have a full length curtain, some have half doors and some a combination of both. It is essential that the shower unit is thermostatically controlled and conforms with British Safety Standards to ensure that clients cannot be scalded if there is a variation in water temperature. The temperature of some showers varies if a person downstairs turns on the cold water tap decreasing the pressure and increasing the heat of the water, clients with limited mobility will not be able to move out of the way quickly. The controls on the shower should be operated easily, a wide range of controls are now available including pushbutton and knobs.

The position from which the client is to shower is also a consideration as, if it is seated, the type of seating provided may influence the choice of cubicle. Shower seats can be:

1. secured to a supporting wall;
2. provided as an integral part of the cubicle;
3. free standing;
4. mobile.

Therapists must determine the most appropriate type for their client, bearing in mind possible weight restrictions of wall-mounted seats and the construction of the wall to which it is to be fixed.

If a client is living in local authority or privately rented accommodation it may not be appropriate to remove the bath permanently. Shower trays are now manufactured to the same dimensions as the bath, provided a showering area and a changing area, and using the same drainage system. When a new tenant moves into the house it is possible to reinstate the bath if required with very little upheaval.

In some situations it may be appropriate to provide an alternative bathroom downstairs and an extension may have to be built. If space is restricted a bathroom cubicle exists which provides a toilet and shower facility within one cubicle requiring very little space. Location will depend upon drainage and situation in relation to the kitchen but for some clients provides a solution to having to move home. A recent addition to the market has been the production of a prefabricated bathroom which can be adjoined to a building. The only preparation needed is the drainage, a concrete base to stand it on and access to the house. The internal design can vary to meet the needs of the individual.

Overhead tracking hoists assist clients with transfers not only into the bath but also on and off of the toilet. They are ceiling fixed and run along either a straight or curved track, used in combination with a sling. In some situations they are installed to assist the carer while in others for the client to use independently. If the client has the upper limb movement to attach the sling to the hoist they can transfer themselves. Slings can be adapted, if necessary to maximize the upper limb function a client has.

Toiletting

The inability to cleanse after using the toilet can be an embarrassing problem for both the client and their carer. The provision of a bidet can overcome this problem and restore dignity and independence for clients. Some bidets have a variety of methods of operation, the most common type used being electrical, and also offer the option of having a warm air drying facility to enable clients to cleanse and dry themselves independently. If a client is dependent upon a carer for toiletting a bidet can greatly assist the carer, as trying to stand someone up, clean them and cope with clothing is extremely difficult.

Mobility problems

Limited mobility can lead to a variety of problems around the house related to:

– access to the house;
– climbing stairs.

Access to the house Access to the house can be a problem not only in terms of the client getting in and out but also in relation to letting visitors in and out. The solution to access problems will inevitably depend upon:

– the client's specific mobility problem;
– the amount of space available leading up to the door.

The main solutions to access problems are:

– lessening the height of the steps;
– providing rails;
– ramping.

If steps are too high for clients to climb doubling the amount of steps halves the height of the step to be taken, this for some clients enables them to gain access more easily. Often the support of rails when climbing steps is beneficial. If a client uses a wheelchair or walking frame the provision of a ramp may be indicated. The recommended gradient for a ramp is 1:20, but this is not always possible, the maximum gradient should be 1:12. If the client's steps lead directly onto a public footpath a permanent ramp cannot be provided as it would obstruct the public highway, in this situation a portable ramp may be more applicable if someone is available to lay it down and remove it after use. The surface of the ramp should be non-slip and a level landing should be provided at the entrance of the house to enable the client to open the door without rolling backwards.

Clients with limited mobility often benefit from the installation of an intercom to enable them to open the front door from their chair. A constant source of frustration to many clients is reaching the door and finding the person has left.

Access to the garage can be a problem as doors are often heavy and require strength and range of movement to open. Automatic doors can provide easy access, by the use of a remote control switch.

Stairs

An adaptation required frequently for clients with rheumatoid disease is the provision of a stair lift to gain access to the upstairs of a house. It is more cost effective than providing a bedroom and bathroom downstairs and is not a permanent feature of the home.

Stairlifts are basically designed with a straight or curved tracking which fits onto the staircase and has a seat which either travels up the stair sideways or backwards. They also provide a footplate. The height of the seat is crucial for many clients, especially in relation to the foot rest as this dictates how much knee flexion is required to sit on the seat and in relation to overall height for transfers on and off of the seat. Stairlifts can also be provided with a standing platform if clients are unable to transfer from a seated position. Some of the seats swivel around so that when the client is getting off at the top of the stairs they can have their back to the staircase and transfer in safety.

The lifts are controlled by a pushbutton switch requiring constant pressure, although alternatives are available for clients with limited hand function, some companies provide rocker switches or joy stick controls.

Throughfloor lifts are provided either where the staircase is unsuitable for the installation of a stairlift or where the client is unable to transfer onto the seat of a stairlift. They are usually situated to travel up into a bedroom. The lift is usually kept upstairs until needed so that it forms part of the ceiling and is brought down into the room when required, enabling the client to walk or wheel in.

This section has covered some of the adaptations that are carried out for clients with rheumatoid disease. Assessment is essential to identify the individual needs of clients and their families and to determine environmental factors which may influence recommendations. Once this has been carried out therapists are then required to identify how these needs can be met within the policy of the particular authority for whom they work. This is often a process of compromise between what is desirable and what is acceptable. Clients must be fully involved in this process to gain an understanding of the processes being gone through and the meaning of this for both themselves, their family and their home.

More clients are now considering paying for adaptations privately, usually due to long waiting lists for assessment or a dissatisfaction with recommendations. The one problem that is encountered by clients, however, is the availability of advice. While some clients may have access to Disabled Living Centres the availability of therapists who can carry out a home visit, which is essential, is limited. Clients in many areas have an all or nothing service whereby the community occupational therapist will assess if an application is made to social services but not if the client wishes to fund the adaptation for themselves. This consultancy service is an area of need which has not been met as yet by the profession and should be addressed.

With the emphasis of healthcare being shifted into the community the need for the provision of both appropriate housing and housing adaptation is essential to ensure that the underlying philosophies of community care become a reality. The environmental barriers provided by a home can be immense resulting in isolation and a dependence upon other people for tasks which, given the right environment, could be carried out independently. The stresses placed upon the family as a whole can develop into a crisis if unrecognized. Clients with rheumatic diseases are not always given high priority on waiting lists as they do not have a life threatening illness nor are they recovering from an acute traumatic event. The problems encountered by clients often fall into low priority categories and can be left for some considerable time before being addressed.

Community care is now a reality and the needs of clients with rheumatoid disease are very much community orientated. The debilitating effect of living in accommodation which is not suitable and does not enable basic needs to be met as independently as possible is substantial, not only on the client but on the whole family unit. Much valuable time and energy can be spent in fulfilling basic needs often leaving clients too tired or in too much pain to consider embarking upon less essential activities. A home which fulfils basic needs is essential to anyone and should be a priority if the potential of community care and integration is to be met, both from the point of view of the client and the whole family unit.

FURTHER READING

E. Bumphrey (1987) *Occupational Therapy in the Community*, Woodhead-Faulkner.

8

Splinting

The fabrication of splints often falls into the remit of therapists working in departments of rheumatology. The types of splints made and materials used vary considerably and it is not the intention of this section to discuss detailed design and fabrication as this is covered comprehensively both in other . publications and the references provided. Before embarking upon the fabrication of splints, therapists must have an understanding of the anatomy of the hand, the structures and their functions and the effects of impairment and splinting upon each. ,

The inflammatory process of rheumatoid disease can affect greatly the stability of joints. Synovial proliferation and effusions stretch and weaken the capsule and ligaments and also erode the cartilage. This process can lead to a laxity of the joint capsule and surrounding structures and hypermobility of the joint leading to subluxation and dislocation. Muscle forces can become altered as they are no longer restricted and alignment may shift leading to an altered direction of pull and abnormal position of the joint. Muscle spasm to protect inflamed joints can lead to deformity and loss of movement, an example of this are the intrinsic muscles of the hand. Tendons can also become inflamed, snap or rupture causing functional loss. Nerve compression can result in functional impairment, loss of sensation and pain, an example of this associated with rheumatoid disease is carpal tunnel syndrome, where the median nerve becomes compressed within the carpal tunnel resulting in numbness and tingling in the first three fingers.

Classification of splints

Splints can be classified either by their design or by their function. Design classification usually refers to a static or dynamic splint. A static splint prevents movement and rests the affected joints. As its primary aim is to immobilize, it should be used as a component of a therapeutic programme to ensure that atrophy, weakness and stiffness do not occur as a result of wearing the splint. If the splint is to be used at home therapists must ensure that the client is aware of the need to exercise an immobilized joint as and when appropriate.

Dynamic splints allow movement and so are constructed to incorporate hinges, elastic or springs or utilize the movement of another body part.

Classification according to the function of the splint falls into three categories:

1. resting;
2. functional;
3. corrective.

These functions are not necessarily mutually exclusive. Their purposes are as follows.

1. Resting splints to:
    - relieve pain;
    - decrease inflammation;
    - prevent the development of contractures;
    - maintain proper hand position;
    - decrease or alleviate symptoms of nerve entrapment;
    - support ligaments and joint capsule.
2. Functional splints to:
    - relieve pain;
    - support unstable structures;
    - accommodate for muscle weakness or atrophy;
    - protect from further damage;
    - assist in controlling inflammation;
    - protect against nerve entrapment or tenosynovitis.
3. Corrective splints to:
    - modify soft tissue contractures (Seeger, 1984).

A further category of splints are those used post-operatively to maintain alignment or mobility, assist with post-operative stretching and minimize adhesions.

Hand assessment

A comprehensive hand assessment must be carried out before a splint is made which not only assesses how the rheumatoid disease has effected the structures of the hand but also its function, these two factors do not necessarily have any correlation. A client with gross deformity may have minimal impairment of hand function whereas a client with minimal deformity may have severe impairment. This is an essential consideration in pre-operative assessment for clients undergoing corrective hand surgery, improvement in alignment does not necessarily lead to an improvement in function.

The process of assessment in relation to splinting aims to:

1. provide baseline measurements against which changes can be documented;
2. identify the priorities, needs and expectations of the client;
3. evaluate the effectiveness of interventions;
4. define the aims and objectives of splinting;
5. identify other interventions which may be appropriate, such as exercise or joint protection.

When assessing the hand it is essential to include an assessment of the wrist, elbow and shoulder as these will all affect the way in which the hand functions and could equally be the cause of pain, loss of movement and loss of function. They can also be affected by the use of splints, for example the weight of splints may have implications for the function of the whole limb and immobilization may also affect other joints. A comprehensive hand assessment includes documentation of the following.

1. The presence of:
   - pain;
   - inflammation;
   - tenderness;
   - oedema;
   - deformity.
2. Range of movement of the:
   - shoulder flexion, extension, abduction, adduction, internal and external rotation;
   - elbow flexion, extension, pronation and supination;
   - wrist flexion, extension, ulnar and radial deviation;

- fingers flexion, extension, adduction and abduction of metacarpalphalangeal joints, proximal and distal phalangeal joints;
- thumb flexion, extension, adduction, abduction, opposition.

It should be noted whether these ranges are of active or passive movement.

1. Grip strength:
   - power grip;
   - pinch grip;
   - cylindrical grip;
   - hook grip.
2. Sensation
3. Function; examples of functional components of assessment include:
   - pouring water from a jug to a glass;
   - writing name;
   - picking up small objects and placing in a container;
   - buttoning and unbuttoning a garment;
   - tying a shoelace;
   - opening and closing a zip;
   - moving different size and shaped objects from one position to another.

In some assessments the functional component is timed or scored. Additional information is needed, as appropriate, about the client's medical condition, and their social situation. The methods for recording the above information will vary depending upon the assessment used. It is essential that a standardized and valid assessment procedure is used and that, as far as is possible, the same therapist carries out each assessment to reduce inter-observer error. Having completed an assessment it is possible to identify the aims and objectives of the splinting programme and the most appropriate type of splint to make.

Fabrication of splints

Having identified the appropriate splint, therapists must then choose the material in which the splint is to be made, design the pattern and then make the splint. There are a wide range of splinting materials on the market most of them comprising thermoplastic materials which become maleable when heat is applied to them, at a variety of temperatures, and resume their rigid state when cooled.

High temperature materials cannot be moulded directly onto the client and therapists need to make a plaster of Paris mould on to which the material can be applied. This process requires several visits to the department as a negative mould is taken first which is then filled with plaster of Paris to provide a positive mould of the client's limb on to which the material can be moulded. Splints produced by this method are usually very resilient and strong, and it is used, therefore, when a splint is required for permanent use, as in a footdrop splint, or is needed to be strong.

The more common splinting materials used are medium and low temperature materials which can be moulded directly onto the client, some requiring a protective layer of gauze, or lubrication between the material and the client's skin. The time taken for the material to cool will vary allowing different working times. Some materials also have the characteristic of memory and when reheated will return to being flat enabling them to be reused, not all materials have memory. Materials become extremely maleable when heated allowing the material to be draped over a limb and moulded into the required shape. Some materials can be moulded utilizing gravity and when draped over a limb will use gravity to attain the desired shape requiring very little moulding on the therapist's behalf. While such material may take a while to become familiar this facility can be beneficial as an excellent fit can be achieved with very little moulding. It does however depend upon the client's ability to maintain the necessary position, i.e. for a foot drop splint clients are required to lie on their stomach, which can be difficult. The materials are heated with either dry or moist heat, and this may dictate choice of material in some working situations.

Plaster of Paris is used less frequently but provides a cheap alternative which is valuable in some situations.

The factors influencing the choice of material include:

1. specific requirement of the splint being made (need to be modified; rigidity; strength; weight; flexibility; size of area being splinted);
2. length of time the splint will be used;
3. speed of which the splint is required;
4. location in which the splint is being made;
5. equipment available;

6. cost of material;
7. skills of the therapist;
8. condition of the client's skin, allergies, open wounds, etc.

Having identified the type of splint and material to be used the next stage is to make the pattern for the splint. Some materials include patterns for standard splints in their packaging and some materials are purchased already cut into standard splint shapes, but these must be checked, if used, on the client for correct fitting. Tracings and measurements are essential to ensure the correct fit of a splint, to avoid pressure areas or boney prominences and to decrease wastage of materials.

When moulding splints directly onto clients therapists must involve the client in the whole procedure. The time taken can be used to pass on information regarding the purpose of the splint, when it is to be used and precautions which may need to be taken. Enabling the client to watch the material being heated is a good way of showing them what will happen if they try to wash it with boiling water or place it near direct heat. Clients should also be reassured about the temperature of the material. It can be frightening to see something being removed from an oven and knowing that it is about to be placed on your hand. Some of the common components of splints for the hand include:

1. transverse metacarpal arch support, supports the anatomical arch;
2. wrist extension bar, stabilizes the wrist;
3. forearm bar, acts as the long lever of the splint;
4. C bar, maintains the web space between thumb and index finger;
5. finger pan, supports all the joints of the fingers, eliminating movement;
6. deviation bar, prevents ulnar or radial deviation;
7. outriggers, extends from the splint to hold dynamic component of splint.

When the splint has been moulded minor alterations may be needed by spot heating. Straps, and if appropriate, padding or lining will be needed. Clients must be able to fit and remove the splint independently and this must be checked. Therapists must also ensure that the client and, if appropriate, nursing staff check the skin for pressure marks after the splint has been worn for a period of time, especially if the splint is dynamic. If there is evidence of pressure marks the splint should be adjusted accordingly.

Splints should be re-evaluated after a period of use to ensure that they are fulfilling the need and that correction or alteration is not needed. Clients must be told how to look after their splint, cleaning methods, when to wear it, appropriate types of exercise to carry out and how to check for pressure problems.

COMMON SPLINTS FOR CLIENTS WITH RHEUMATOID DISEASE

Resting splint

This splint is designed to extend from the mid forearm to the tips of the fingers, supporting the palmar aspect of the hand. It is used to maintain the hand in a functional position providing rest to the joints and decreasing inflammation.

The splints are fabricated with varying degrees of wrist extension which should not exceed 30°, and should be within a painfree range. If a client has carpal tunnel syndrome the wrist should be maintained in a neutral position. The fingers are slightly flexed. An ulnar ridge may be needed if clients have ulnar deviation to maintain the fingers in the correct alignment. The thumb is opposed and abducted.

Functional wrist splint

This splint is frequently used to immobilize the wrist during activity ensuring that the MCPs and the thumb can still be used unobstructed. Clients often find the support beneficial when carrying out activities of daily living.

To ensure unobstructed use of the hand the splint should not extend, on the palmar aspect of the hand, beyond the proximal palmar crease and must also allow a cutout around the thenar eminence. The splint extends up to the mid forearm. These splints are often made commercially with strong stretch elastic material and a reinforced brace extending from the palmar crease down over the wrist to the forearm, on the palmar aspect. However, as they are usually provided in standard sizes the fit must be checked. Clients are often present with ill-fitting splints which impair their hand function, usually because they extend beyond the proximal palmar crease.

Corrective splints

One form of corrective splint used in conjunction with a programme of physiotherapy is a back slab which is used for clients who have developed reversible knee contractures. They are used to maintain stretch gained therapeutically and are usually applied after physiotherapy. The position of the splint must be altered frequently to ensure that it is maintaining the increased extension achieved during treatment.

Corrective splints are used to re-align fingers and overcome functional problems created by ulnar drift.

Splints are always used as a component of a therapeutic programme which includes, not only assessment of the hand but evaluation of the effectiveness of the splint in improving range of movement or function, decreasing pain or preventing or improving deformity. Splints should be used in conjunction with exercise, and assessment may also indicate the need for education in relation to joint protection or energy conservation.

FURTHER READING

N. Barr (1975) *The Principles and Techniques of Simple Splint Making in Rehabilitation*, Butterworth, Guildford.

R. Cailliet (1982) *Hand Pain and Impairment*, 3rd edn, F.A. Davis Company.

Fess and Philips (1987) *Hand Splinting Principles and Methods*, 2nd edn, The C.V. Mosby Company, St Louis.

C. Moran (1986) *Hand Rehabilitation*, Churchill Livingstone, London.

9

Relaxation and pain control

Pain is the most predominant symptom of rheumatoid disease and the most frequent reason for seeking medical assistance. The most common form of pain relief for clients with rheumatoid disease is the prescription of analgesia. Many clients, however, express concern about the long term implications of prolonged use of analgesia and seek alternative methods of control. Some of these have been discussed already, the use of heat and ice and joint protection, others extend into the field of complimentary medicine. It is now acknowledged widely that the explanation and definition of pain is a complex issue which is no longer sought purely on the basis of a physiological cause. Recent theories of pain have acknowledged the fact that they must account for:

1. the high degree of physiological specialization of receptor–fibre units and of pathways in the central nervous system;
2. the role of temporal and spatial patterning in the transmission of information in the central nervous system;
3. the influence of psychological processes on pain perception and response;
4. the clinical phenomena of spatial and temporal summation, spread of pain and persistence of pain after healing (Melzack, 1982).

This multi-dimensional approach is evident in the management of pain. Pain clinics are establishing management approaches which include the use of drugs, behaviour modification, relaxation, biofeedback, exercise and activity. Approaches vary considerably but it is now apparent that the skills of paramedics are important in helping clients to manage their pain.

The experience of pain, as has already been stated, is subjective and as such is difficult for clients to explain and clinicians to measure. As one client said, 'I hate it when my doctor asks if I am in pain because if I say yes I know he will ask me to describe it and it is impossible'; the word ache or stabbing or burning can mean so many different things and the way in which they are interpreted will vary also. The subjective nature of pain means that everyone will experience and react to it in different ways. Many factors other than an underlying pathology can influence the experience of pain, including the amount of attention paid to the pain, previous experiences of pain and observation of the reaction of other people to pain, not only in relation to the client but those around them.

The way in which a parent responds to a child who falls over or knocks themselves serves to reinforce behaviour, as does the way children observe their parents reacting to pain. Many clients will relate how sleeping is a problem because pain seems worse during the night often the basis for this is that there is no distraction and attention focuses solely on the pain increasing its perceived intensity.

A person's perceived ability to cope with their rheumatoid disease can also affect their perception of the pain they are experiencing, for example, a client with active disease may be functioning relatively well at home until a crisis occurs in the home and then the pain they are experiencing can increase and their coping ability decrease. The disease activity does not alter necessarily but their ability to cope with the perceived increase in pain has. The reverse is also true as well, on a day to day basis, if a client has something to achieve they will work through their pain to achieve it and will often relate how the pain they experienced was reduced, especially if the activity is highly valued or absorbing. The extreme examples of the scope of psychological interventions to control pain are the operations which have been performed, and televised, without the use of anaesthetics as a result of using hypnosis, or the rituals practised in some cultures during religious festivals.

Behavioural therapists refer to 'pain related behaviour' which some clients have evolved and can be reinforced by interaction with society and the family, often unintentionally. When a person is experiencing acute pain recognition is given to the pain by others and allowances made, when the pain is chronic other people's reaction will change over a period of time and recognition may be lost unless it is actively sought. Attention can be drawn to the pain a client may be experiencing by grimacing, wincing and complaining and can have the desired effect of drawing attention and gaining sympathy, avoiding doing specific tasks or receiving medication. A behavioural approach to pain-related behaviour is to replace the negative pain behaviour with more positive responses, teaching the client to approach their pain in a positive way rather than constantly seeking empathy, sympathy and concern. Comprehensive programmes are available which serve to modify pain related behaviour and reinforce more appropriate responses conveying other positive coping strategies, such as exercise, relaxation and bio-feedback. Some of these programmes also aim to reduce the amount of medication a client is taking. Three questions have been raised in relation to such programmes.

1. Does the patient actually feel less pain or have they simply learnt to complain less?
2. How do the programmes compare to the placebo effect? Such programmes usually necessitate constant attention and hospital admission.
3. Such programmes are expensive to implement and run and if the programmes are effective will they be available to everyone? (Melzack, 1982)

Most clients with rheumatoid disease will experience a variety of different types and intensities of pain. The pain may be acute, as during a flare or as the result of an infected joint, or chronic, a background pain which is present for much of the time. Total pain relief is something which most clients do not experience, the medication they take usually brings the pain down to a level at which it can be tolerated and activities carried out, there is still often a background pain. The most obvious source of pain for clients with rheumatoid disease is the inflammatory process occurring in their joints but the multi-systemic nature of rheumatoid disease can lead to pain arising from a variety of different sources:

1. referred pain, hip pain can be referred to the thigh muscles;
2. pain arising from nerve entrapment or compression, as in carpal tunnel syndrome;
3. pain arising from vascular disease, as in Raynauds Disease or as a result of vasculitis;
4. pain resulting from surgical procedures. The pain experienced following a knee replacement can be intense and needs to be well controlled to enable therapy to commence.

The treatment of pain in relation to rheumatoid disease can be categorized as follows:

1. cutaneous stimulation, i.e. massage, to relieve spasm and tension;

2. thermal modalities, heat, ice or a combination of both;
3. transcutaneous electrical nerve stimulation (TENS);
4. pharmacological;
5. relaxation techniques;
6. rest;
7. mechanical methods such as traction (Smith-Pigg, 1985).

The way in which rest and joint protection can be used to reduce pain have already been discussed but an area not previously covered is the use of relaxation techniques. Most techniques require very little equipment, other than a quiet room with comfortable chairs or floor mats, and can be used easily at home. They aim to reduce muscle tension, lower the heart rate, respiratory rate and blood pressure and help clients cope with stress which is present when coping with rheumatoid disease. Before embarking upon relaxation sessions it is essential that clients understand the rationale behind the use of the technique and the expected outcome. Emphasis should also be placed upon the fact that relaxation is a skill which can be learnt and that it may take several sessions for a relaxed state to be achieved.

Relaxation sessions should be carried out in an environment which is free from distraction (something which can be difficult in a busy hospital setting) warm and comfortable. Some clients will be unable to lie on the floor and will be more comfortable sitting in a chair but it should provide good head and arm support and be the correct height. The use of foot stools may provide more comfort.

The most common types of relaxation used in a clinical setting are:

1. guided imagery and visualization;
2. progressive muscle relaxation;
3. controlled rhythmic breathing;
4. biofeedback;
5. yoga.

Guided imagery

This method entails evoking images of relaxation, calm and peaceful situations. Therapists usually provide an introduction focusing the client's attention on their breathing and muscles, taking deep breaths and feeling the weight of their limbs. Clients are then slowly introduced to a setting such as a beach drenched with the warmth of the sun, being in a meadow or wood or gliding and drifting in the sky. Having built up some of the imagery around the situation clients are then allowed time to develop their own imagery further before being brought back to the room in which the session is being held. Some therapists use music to add to the imagery and evoke a relevant mood. However some people feel this can be intrusive as peoples' taste in music varies so much that it could be a distraction.

Autogenic techniques can also be used in conjunction with this technique by asking clients to feel the warmth of the sun on their body or the heaviness of their limbs. Clients should be encouraged to develop their own imagery and take themselves to a place which, for them, is identified with calm and peace. Visualization is very similar to guided imagery but clients are asked to visualize tension and pain leaving their body, so the pain may be visualized and placed into an object which is watched moving away.

Progressive muscle relaxation

This method concentrates on specific muscle groups working through the body tensing and relaxing them. Usually the programme begins with the feet and works up the body. Muscles are tensed while inhaling and relaxed while exhaling. The advantage of this technique is that it provides a contrast between tension and relaxation enabling clients to distinguish between the two. The disadvantage is that some clients may find that tensing muscle groups elicits pain and discomfort in which case the benefits of the relaxation will be lost.

Controlled breathing

This method focuses directly on lowering the respiratory rate by asking clients to concentrate on their breathing taking deeper breaths in and slowly exhaling. Sometimes a word is used as a focus on exhaling such as 'peace' or 'calm'.

Biofeedback

Biofeedback provides an excellent visual feedback for a client on their ability to control heart rate, muscle tension, blood pressure or body temperature. A simple form of biofeedback utilizes a small hand-held thermometer. As the client becomes more relaxed the temperature increases. Electronic feedback can also be provided by the use of monitors enabling the client to see how using a relaxation technique, for example, lowers their heart rate or reduces tension in muscles. They can be shown read-outs for a state of muscle tension and muscle relaxation and learn how to develop their relaxation skills to achieve a relaxed state and influence the readings. Biofeedback provides the client with specific information about their ability to influence their body and also enables the distinction to be made between a state of relaxation and tension.

Yoga

When yoga is suggested to many clients they have visions of being twisted and contorted into strange positions or of being asked to achieve the lotus position. However, participating in yoga classes can enable clients to learn controlled breathing techniques, relaxation techniques and good posture. This combination of relaxation, attention to posture and controlled exercise may be beneficial to many clients. As has already been stated pain and discomfort can lead to a flexed posture, round shoulders and muscle tension, it can also impair respiration and so attention not only to tension but also to posture can be beneficial. With the growing popularity of yoga some instructors are now extending their training to develop the skills necessary to teach yoga to people with a physical disability. While the above techniques can be used in the quiet of the home, yoga is an activity which is carried out in many recreation centres or as a component of adult education courses and so has the added benefit of social contact.

Relaxation is a coping strategy which can be presented to clients as a method of pain control and of coping with the effects of stress. It is not seen as something which is different or obscure as it is a popular means of dealing with stress, tension and pain which is well publicized in the popular press and on television. It is inexpensive and is easily carried out at home, either during the day or night. It can be used for five minutes or half an hour depending on the technique being used. One of the factors contributing to the experience of pain is a feeling of not being in control of it. Relaxation is a method for gaining some control back and is used not only to deal with pain but also the stress, anxiety and tension that can result from living with rheumatoid disease.

FURTHER READING

Dr R. Sternbach (1987) *Mastering Pain*, Arlington Books.

10

Personal and sexual relationships

Personal and sexual relationships can be affected profoundly by the onset or progression of a chronic disease. This can be due either to the physical symptoms of pain, stiffness, limitation of movement and fatigue or the psychological impact of the disease which can effect a person's sexuality by lowering self-esteem, leading to a decreased interest in sexual activities as a result of stress, anxiety and depression, or changes in body image can lead to a client to perceive themselves as unattractive. Social contact may be decreased by any of the above factors limiting opportunities to meet potential partners.

Problems can also arise due to a partner's fear of causing pain or damage to a joint, their increased fatigue due to an increase of workload and having to take on extra responsibilities. It may also take partners a while to come to terms with the onset of deformities and the way in which their partner is changing bodily.

This potential problem area should be considered with clients regardless of age or whether the client is married, in a stable relationship or single. The ways in which a chronic disease can affect sexuality have already been discussed and emphasis placed upon the fact that sexual function can not be considered purely in relation to the mechanical act of sexual intercourse but must be considered in relation to sexuality as well. Some of the issues which therapists need to consider in relation to personal and sexual relationships are the communication of information to the client and if appropriate their partner, concepts of sexuality and sexual fulfilment, practical advice and contraception.

Communication

The issue of communication needs to be considered both in relation to communication between therapist and client and between partners.

The communication of information regarding personal and sexual relationships between therapists and clients is often an area of concern for both people. In many instances the topic is omitted from routine assessment and the onus is then placed upon the client to draw any problems to the attention of the therapist. The outcome of this is that sexual problems frequently remain unexpressed.

Reasons for this are related usually to therapists feeling unable to deal with problems if they are expressed and questioning their own ability to cope with this issue. It is necessary to consider, however, the implications of not acknowledging the sexuality of a client and the messages implicit in avoidance of the subject. It may serve to reinforce a client's feeling of becoming asexual and unattractive and lead to suppression of a lot of anxiety and stress. 'They feel I am past it' is an unspoken message which can be conveyed.

Communication between partners is essential to cope with the changes in their sexual relationship which may be occurring. The ease of communication will to some extent depend upon how the couple communicated regarding their sexual relationship before the onset of rheumatoid disease. If it was a subject which was never discussed, facing changes and overcoming problems may be difficult for both partners and they may need some assistance in addressing any problems which arise. The progression of the disease may lead to a need to change the way in which sexual feelings are expressed and for both partners to consider alternative ways of providing pleasure for each other. In any relationship when this occurs partners need to feel confident with each other to explore alternative methods and not feel pressurized into participating in something they feel uncomfortable with. The needs of both partners have to be considered and alternatives found which they both feel happy with.

Experimentation of new positions or new ways of providing pleasure may identify dislikes as well as likes and new methods may not work at first. In this situation the ability to discuss any problems which may have arisen or the fact that one partner was not happy with what occurred, without feeling a sense of failure is essential. It is easy for one failure to place pressure upon clients the next time they have intercourse leading to tension in the female which can cause pain and discomfort during intercourse and inability to attain or maintain an erection for the male. This pressure in itself can exacerbate problems and make sexual functioning more difficult. The majority of clients referred to sex therapists have psychological rather than physical problems which interfere with their sexual functioning. If clients do express sexual difficulties assumptions should not be made that these are due to purely physical reasons.

Concepts of sexual fulfilment

Concepts of sexual fulfilment differ greatly but are equated frequently to sexual intercourse. However many people participate in sexually fulfilling relationships using a whole range of sexual expression which includes attention to sensuality as well as sexual intercourse. The environment, comfort, and the use of pleasuring are all important components of a sexual relationship and the method by which an orgasm is attained does not necessarily have to be via penetration of the penis into the vagina.

When sexual relationships are discussed it is easy for attention to be paid to penetrative sex and for other means of sexual expression to be ignored. Limitation in movement can mean that penetrative sex is difficult or painful and that alternatives need to be found. This may include oral sex or the use of vibrators or other sex aids, or experimentation with different positions.

Partners who have always been used to penetrative sex and have not experimented very much in their sexual relationship may feel anxious about change. They may feel that some of the alternatives are perceived as being 'kinky' or approaching the boundaries of normal sexual relationships. This needs to be established in discussion by the therapist so that suggestions are not made in an inappropriate way that may shock or offend the client or their partner. In such circumstances discussion and reassurance can relieve a lot of anxiety.

It is essential to remember that the sexual response is unlearned but that sexual behaviour is learned. The extent of peoples' sex education is extremely variable and assumptions should not be made that clients are familiar with the terminology being used or that their understanding of phrases is the same as yours. If, as a small group exercise, a list was drawn up of all the names which are used to describe either sexual organs or sexual intercourse the margin for misconceptions to occur would be seen to be great. Therapists should ensure that the language they use is the same as the client and adapt their own terminology accordingly.

Many images and expectations of sexual relationships and activity are learnt from the media. The stereotypical relationship is of an earth moving and multiple orgasmic experience for both partners.

Clients should be reassured that the important factor is what they find mutually fulfilling and are both happy with: there is no such thing as a 'normal' sexual relationship.

Practical advice

Some of the problems encountered by clients are associated with aspects of sexuality and personal relationships which may be resolved by counselling, either for the client or the client and their partner. Other problems may be dealt with by access to practical information and advice. Often a combination of both may be required.

Improving self-image is an issue which can be addressed with clients. Outward appearance can affect the entire way in which we function in society and the non-verbal messages which are conveyed. When a person embarks upon a new personal relationship or is feeling good about the way they look people pick up these messages without any verbal prompting. Confidence in appearance can affect the gait, posture and communication. While counselling can help a client come to terms with changes in body image, time can also be spent helping a client to make the most of their assets. A change in make-up, clothes and hairstyle can all boost a person's confidence and self-esteem which is usually conveyed in social interactions. It is easy for everyone to point out their limitations and more difficult to sit down and consider assets and ways in which these can be capitalized upon. Such activities are an ideal topic for groups to address as the sharing process can provide support and confidence. Enhancing aspects of a person's appearance can draw attention away from deformities, posture or gait.

Pain and stiffness can interfere with sexual activities and ways in which these can be alleviated may need to be considered. It is sometimes necessary to give thought to the timing of sexual intercourse, identifying the best time of the day or planning to take meditation beforehand. A warm bath or shower may also help to relieve pain and stiffness as may massage. These can be incorporated as part of making love.

Finding a comfortable position is often a question of partners being creative and experimenting. Male clients may seek positions which do not require bearing all their body weight through their arms and legs and women may seek positions in which they are not required to externally rotate or flex their hips and knees to a great degree or bear a lot of weight.

Cushions and pillows can be used to provide support and padding. The systemic effects of rheumatoid disease can lead to decreased vaginal secretions and clients may need to use a lubricant to make entry into the vagina more comfortable.

In some situations penetrative sex may be too difficult and other methods of providing sexual satisfaction needed. Masturbation is one way of achieving an orgasm for couples or people who are not involved in a relationship. If a client's hands are affected the aid of a vibrator may be required. Oral sex is another way of providing pleasure for a partner and positions can be found which are comfortable and place no pressure upon painful joints.

There are several publications which graphically describe aspects of sexual relationships and cover topics such as pleasuring, different positions and communication. They are widely available in bookshops and do not have a special emphasis on sexual relationships for people with disabilities. Mail order catalogues can be used to purchase a whole variety of sex aids as many sex shops are inaccessible.

It is also worth remembering that some medication can decrease a person's libido and also contribute to men not being able to attain an erection. While some clients may only need access to information others may be experiencing a more complex problem and require counselling or sex therapy.

Contraception

Clients with limited manual dexterity may be experiencing difficulties in using some forms of contraception. A diaphragm, especially when coated with a spermicidal jelly, can be slippery and difficult to hold and insert. Men may experience similar difficulties using a condom, but partners can assist. While intra-uterine devices do not present problems in insertion they may present problems for some women in coping with heavier periods which may be a result of use. Some of the non-steroidal anti-inflammatory drugs and other medication which may be prescribed can affect the effectiveness of birth control pills. Clients should be advised to check with their doctor if they think this may be a problem.

Advice regarding sexual relationships may be required following joint replacement surgery. A person having undergone a total hip arthroplasty will need guidance as to when they can resume previous levels of sexual activity. The length of time during which surgeons wish clients to refrain from sexual intercourse varies and should be confirmed with individual surgeons.

To enable clients to discuss sexual and personal relationships, therapists should include this aspect of function in routine functional assessments. As assessments include elements relating to personal hygiene and cover cleansing after using the toilet or the use of sanitary protection, sexual activity fits into this area of assessment without appearing false. In a clinic, ward or department literature can be left easily accessible so that clients will know that this is a subject which is open for discussion if they should so wish. In view of the courage it takes to initiate discussion on this topic it is correct to place the onus upon the therapist to provide an atmosphere in which sexual problems can be discussed freely if the client wishes. If a therapist feels unable to deal with these problems they must inform themselves of other colleagues within the team or within other agencies who are willing to see clients in relation to sexual problems.

Consideration should be given to the way in which clients are referred on to colleagues or other agencies. One client seen in an out-patient clinic expressed problems she was having in her sexual relationship and was immediately told 'I think you should go and see. . .'. She was not given an opportunity to discuss her problems in a generalized way and felt that her trust had been betrayed. She never did go to the outside agency as she had never heard of it, did not know where it was and did not feel able to discuss her problem with a total stranger. The experience reinforced the fact that sexual relationships were not a subject to discuss. The reaction she received was an outward expression of an inward panic felt by many professionals when sexual relationships are brought up in discussion. It is interesting to examine the attitudes, prejudices and feelings which are expressed when the reasons behind such responses are explored with groups of professionals. There is no reason why everyone should feel able to deal with client's sexual problems but everyone should be able to acknowledge a client's sexuality and possible need of assistance in this area and be able to refer to it in a way which is sensitive and ensures that the client's problem is not purely suppressed.

FURTHER READING

W. Greengross (1976) *Entitled to Love, The Sexual and Emotional Needs of the Handicapped*, Malaby Press.

W. Stewart (1979) *The Sexual Side of Handicap, A Guide for the Caring Professions*, Woodhead-Faulkner.

11

Community care

The topic of community care is an extremely pertinent issue in relation to both the management of rheumatoid disease and the changing emphasis of healthcare from a hospital into a community setting. The underlying philosophies and objectives of community care are central to the management of rheumatoid disease, which while managed clinically in a hospital setting, is predominantly a community issue. As has been shown throughout the preceding chapters while the underlying disease process causes impairment it is far from the only cause of disability and handicap. The nature and level of support available to the client and their carers, access to information, resources and facilities in relation to education, employment and recreation, and the availability of appropriate housing will all affect greatly the quality of life for clients with rheumatoid disease. Most of these, it is argued, depend upon the availability of funds but the way in which resources are used and the attitudes, values and policies of those who control them is crucial.

The way in which resources are being used is a topic of increasing concern not only amongst government and management circles but also amongst people with disabilities who are no longer prepared to play a passive role in relation to issues which have major implications on the way in which they live their life. This changing climate has been set against almost a decade of reports, reviews and legislation relating to the practice of healthcare and changes in social policy. The major contributions have been made by:

1981 *Care in Action*. A Handbook of Policies for the Health and Personal Social Services in England;

1985 *Living Options*. Guidelines for those Planning Services for People with Severe Physical Disabilities;

1986 *Physical Disabilities in 1986 and Beyond*. Report of the Royal College of Physicians;

1986 *Review of Artificial Limb and Appliance Centre Services.* McColl Report;

1986 Disabled Persons (Services, Consultation and Representation) Act;

1988 *Last on the List.* Community Services for People with a Physical Disability, Kings Fund Institute Report;

1988 *Living Options Lottery.* Housing and Support Services for People with Physical Disabilities. The Princes of Wales' Advisory Group on Disability;

1988 *Community Care.* An Agenda for Action;

1988 *A Positive Choice.* Report of the Independent Review of Residential Care;

1989 *Working for Patients.* Government White Paper;

1989 *Caring for People.* Community Care in the Next Decade and Beyond. Government White Paper.

The picture painted of the state of existing services by the majority of the above reports and reviews is extremely bleak raising many issues relating to the services and provision for clients with a chronic disability between the ages of 16–65 years. One of the issues which is raised several times is that while there has been a development of services for people with a mental illness, mental handicap or for the elderly, services for clients falling into the young chronic sick age group have fallen behind. This is not to say that services for the other three groups are satisfactory. It is necessary to define community care before embarking upon a closer examination of some of the issues raised. The DHSS definition of community care states that it is:

a matter of marshalling resources, sharing responsibilities and combining skills to achieve good quality modern services to meet the actual needs of real people in the ways those people find acceptable and in places which encourage rather than prevent normal living.

The principles are defined precisely as:

- to enable an individual to remain in his own home, wherever possible, rather than being cared for in a hospital or residential home;
- to give support and relief to informal carers (family, friends and neighbours) coping with the stress of caring for a dependent person;

185

- to deliver appropriate help, by the means which cause the least possible disruption to ordinary living;
- to relieve the stresses and strains contributing to or arising from physical or emotional disorder;
- to provide the most cost effective package of services to meet the needs and wishes of those being helped;
- to integrate all the resources of a geographical area in order to support the individuals within it.

This was expanded to include 'the need for assessment of the individual in his or her own situation, taking account of all the resources that may be available and the gap which may exist between the assistance those resources provide and the individual's needs' and the preventative and rehabilitative role of community care.

Throughout the legislature and government reviews the role of the statutory services has been identified as supporting existing social networks this was made clear in a statement to the House of Commons:

> The great bulk of community care will continue to be provided by family, friends and neighbours. The majority of carers take on these responsibilities willingly and I admire the dedicated and self-sacrificing way in which so many members of the public take on serious obligations to help care for elderly or disabled relatives and friends. Our proposals are aimed at strengthening support for those many unselfish people who care for people in need (Clarke, 1989).

This view is not necessarily one shared by groups representing people with disabilities. The demands made upon carers and families can be huge and a continuing debate is whether it is acceptable to withhold statutory support from clients with husbands/wives or teenage children. One client was extremely upset when she was told that she could not receive home help because she had teenage children living at home with her. Her constant question was 'why should my children be penalized by my disability?' Therapists are constantly confronted with such questions which are often difficult to answer. This issue has also cropped up with a client with rheumatoid disease who had been receiving support services until he was married and then they were withdrawn.

The consistent picture which has emerged of community services is one of fragmentation, huge discrepancies in service provision and lack of co-ordination within a system which does not consistently seek to establish client needs or respond to them and from a users point of view a system about which there is little information and from which there is little consultation. Similar criticisms have also been made in relation to rehabilitation services. The main type of support clients need is in relation to social support. Social support services include:

1. personal assistance;
2. household management;
3. special housing;
4. aids and equipment;
5. day care;
6. respite for carers;
7. counselling and advice (Beardshaw, 1988).

The need for flexible personal support services is expressed frequently by clients with rheumatoid disease. The condition itself is variable and this may mean that variable amounts of support are required. During an exacerbation more frequent help may be needed, or help of a different kind. In some areas this flexibility is being increased by the introduction of domiciliary care attendants whose remit is far wider than home helps including personal assistance as well as household chores.

This generic approach to care also serves to reduce the number of people calling to assist one client. The total number of support workers calling on one house can be large making it more difficult for individuals to get to know the needs of the client, which can be complex in some cases. The amount of communication between services and agencies is seen as minimal leading to a fragmented approach.

There is an acute lack of special housing in many areas, with waiting lists being immense. A similar picture is painted for the provision of equipment and housing adaptations. The time that clients have to wait is too long and the service with which they are provided falls short, often, of their expectations. The supply of equipment is made more complicated by the number of agencies involved. In some areas joint finance is used to provide a centrally co-ordinated equipment store but other areas still have distinctions between equipment supplied by the health service, usually commodes and nursing consumables, and equipment provided by social services. This system is confusing for clients and professionals.

Access to day-care for clients in this younger group is minimal, compared to other priority groups, as is the availability of respite care. One fact that has also been raised is that clients tend to receive services when they reach a crisis point and cannot carry on as they have been doing.

Clients are not sure how the system works and are frequently disappointed when their expectations of what they perceive to be the system is not met. Clients are not always told when their case has been closed and do not understand the implications of what this may mean. Clients are frequently met who cannot understand why the therapist or social worker has not called to see them for over a year and are unaware that they have to re-refer themselves if a subsequent problem arises. Many clients have the expectation that once in contact with social services that contact will continue. Lack of information and communication is one of the most frequent causes of dissatisfaction and distress.

While some of the issues raised can be seen as a result of inadequate levels of provision and funding many others are reflective of working practices of the service providers. Perhaps these issues are raised even less because of the personal implications for professionals, '. . . these include problems of communication with clients and poor co-ordination with other professionals, which combine with rigid approaches to treatment to result in a general failure to adapt interventions to individual needs.' This problem is seen not only in relation to social support services but also primary health care and disability services. The responsibility for changing working practices can be off loaded onto higher levels of management or onto the availability of resources, but the bottom line is that it also starts with the practice, attitudes and skills of healthcare professionals like occupational therapists.

Community care is a much greater issue than service provision and encompasses full integration into all aspects of community life, participation in the identification of needs and the planning of services and personal choice. Therapists may feel that these issues are only of relevance to management but this is not the case. The following principles can be applied throughout the whole structure of healthcare.

Choice

As to where to live and how to maintain independence without overprotection, or the risk of unnecessary hazards. This includes help in learning how to choose from the options available – a skill that needs to be acquired from an early age.

Consultation

On services as they are planned and knowledge that such services will be based on the views of people with disability, their carers' families and voluntary organizations with special expertise. Particular note should be taken of the views of those from differing cultural backgrounds.

Information

Clearly presented and readily available to the most severely disabled consumers and their families, these service providers and those responsible for planning.

Participation

In the life of local and national communities in respect of both responsibilities and benefits. Full integration can only exist when equal opportunities are available in the fields of access, housing, employment, education, mobility and leisure.

Recognition

That long-term disability is not synonymous with illness and that the medical model of care is inappropriate in the majority of cases.

Autonomy

That is, freedom to make decisions regarding the way of life best suited to an individual disabled person's circumstances (Fielder, 1988).

These guidelines should be fundamental to the planning and execution of any service related to people with rheumatoid disease and an honest examination of both personal practice and the functioning of a team or department with these in mind is often a salutary experience.

Clients do not have such a degree of social mobility if they need housing adaptations when they move. How much consultation is carried out on the type of equipment purchased by a social services department? The decisions are usually taken purely on a financial basis with little evaluation about the effectiveness or the performance, by people who very rarely use equipment. Clients often have strong opinions regarding the equipment they use every day but are consulted rarely. Their experience and contribution is a valuable learning process for any therapist who may have a totally different concept of the equipment.

There is often little choice about the type of care a client receives and when it is given. Support services are inflexible and not always available when the client needs them. Clients needing assistance going to bed may receive nursing services any time from 7.00pm onwards due to pressure of work. Examples do exist where clients have individual choice being given the money by a local authority to purchase their own care as and when required, these situations usually arise as a result of determination on the client's behalf or a forward thinking authority and shows that it is possible for obstacles to be removed.

Another key element to choice is the emphasis on the fact that choosing options is a skill. It is not enough to merely present choices to clients without explaining the options and the implications. Clients are often outside the system, do not know how it works or have access to all the information that professionals have and this imbalance must be redressed if choice is to become a reality. Disability forums are emerging as are other representative groups in many local areas and such groups should be given assistance to learn skills related to chairing meetings, taking minutes, speaking in public and so on. Professionals have access to numerous training days to learn such skills and these opportunities should be available to clients to enable them to contribute in a meaningful way in consultation procedures.

Choice, consultation and participation are all reliant upon access to information and access in its widest sense of physical access to buildings where the information is kept and access in terms of the presentation of information in an appropriate format. Information should not only be available to clients but also to healthcare professionals who find the systems, policies and procedures as confusing. There is a need for a greater understanding of different professional roles and a sharing of information in team situations. This becomes even more important when information needs to cross from a hospital setting into the community. The larger the team the more difficult communication of information becomes, but unless this happens a planned approach to management is difficult with people aiming for different goals.

The above principles are not seen as an idealistic utopia, they can become a reality even within a climate of financial constraint and cut-backs. While the provision of services and housing at realistic levels may need finance, the availability of which is usually a political question, choice, consultation, information, participation, recognition and autonomy largely relate to attitudes, philosophies and working practice. The bar to them, all too frequently, is the attitudes of professionals who conform to a system without questioning the rationale behind policies and procedures accepting them as tablets of stone which cannot be changed.

One of the challenges and frustrations of working with clients with rheumatoid disease is the enormous number of questions which remain unanswered. This challenge has led many therapists into research to try and find answers to specific questions and has likewise led therapists into examining their practices of work. It is hoped that as long as questions are being asked of and from therapists their contribution to the management of rheumatoid disease will develop, providing a service which seeks to identify and respond to the needs of clients and their carers and maintains the client as the central component of the team, not merely as a recipient of treatment and information, but as the focus.

FURTHER READING

V. Beardshaw (1988) *Last on the List, Community Services for People with Physical Disabilities*, Kings Fund Institute, London.

M. Bulmar (1987) *The Social Basis of Community Care*, Unwin Hyman.

B. Fiedler *Living Options Lottery, Housing and Support Services for People with Severe Physical Disabilities, 186/88*, The Prince of Wales Advisory Group on Disability.

C. Hicks (1988) *Who Cares? Looking After People at Home*, Virago Press, London.

References

Anderson, K., Bradley, C., Young, L. and McDaniel, L. (1985) Rheumatoid arthritis: review of psychological factors related to aetiology, effects and treatment, *Psychological Bulletin*, **98** (2) 358–87.

Arthritis and Rheumatism Council Information Booklets, Arthritis and Rheumatism Council, 41 Eagle Street, London.

Arthritis and Rheumatism Council Booklet, *Are You Sitting Comfortably?*, ARC, 41 Eagle Street, London.

Baum, J. (1982) A review of the psychological aspects of rheumatic diseases, *Seminars in Arthritis and Rheumatism*, **11** (3), 352–61.

Beardshaw, V. (1988) *Last on the List, Community Services for People with Physical Disabilities*, Kings Fund Institute.

Brattstromm, M. (1987) *Joint Protection and Rehabilitation in Chronic Rheumatic Disorders*, 3rd edn, Wolfe Medical Publications Ltd, London.

Breakwell, G. (1986) *Coping With Threatened Identities*, Methuen, London.

Burnard, P. (1989) *Counselling Skills for Health Professionals*, Therapy in Practice No. 9, Chapman and Hall, London, pp. 88–96.

Chronically Sick and Disabled Persons Act, 1970.

Clarke, K. (1989) Statement to Parliament.

Cohen, F. and Lazarus, R. (1979) Coping with the stresses of illness, in *Health Psychology: A Handbook* (eds G.C. Stone, F. Cohen and N.E. Adler), Josey Bass, San Francisco.

Cordery, J.C. (1965) Joint protection a responsibility of the occupational therapist, *American Journal of Occupational Therapy*, **19**, 285–94.

Cox, T. (1978) *Stress*, Macmillan Education, London, p. 25.

DHSS (1984–5) *Government response to the second report from the social services committee*, community care.

DHSS (1984–5) Evidence to the House of Commons Committee on Social Services (HC13).

DHSS, Equipment Evaluation Programme.

Disabled Living Foundation Equipment Lists, Disabled Living Foundation, 380–4 Harrow Road, London, W9 2HU.

Disabled Persons (Services, Consultation and Representation) Act, 1986.

Eakin, P. (1989) Problems of Assessments of Activities of Daily Living, *British Journal of Occupational Therapy*, **52** (2), 50–4 and pp. 11–15.

Equipment for Disabled People Series, Mary Marlborough Lodge, Nuffield Orthopaedic Centre, Oxford, OX3 7LD.

Ferguson, K. and Boyle, G. (1978) Family support, health beliefs and therapeutic compliance in patients with rheumatoid arthritis, *Patient Counselling and Health Education*, Winter/Spring pp. 101–5.

Fielder, B. (1988) *Living Options Lottery*, The Prince of Wales Advisory Group on Disability.

Fries, J., Spitz, P., Kraines, G. and Holman, H. (1980) Measurement of Patient Outcome in Arthritis, *Arthritis and Rheumatism*, **23** (2), 137–45.

Furst, G., Gerber, L. and Smith, C. (1982) *Rehabilitation Through Learning: Energy Conservation and Joint Protection. A Workbook for Persons with Rheumatoid Arthritis*, US Department of Health and Human Services.

Griffiths, R. (1988) *Community Care: Agenda for Action*, DHSS.

Halpern, A. and Fuhrer, M. (1984) *Functional Assessment in Rehabilitation*, P.H. Brookes Publishing Company, Baltimore.

Hayward, A. and Sparks, J. (1986) *The Concise English Dictionary*, Omega Books, Herts.

Kaye, R. and Hammond, A. (1978) Understanding Rheumatoid Arthritis, *Journal of the American Medical Association*, **239** (23), 2466–7.

Kelman, H. and Willner, A. (1962) Problems in Measurement and Evaluation of Rehabilitation, *Archives of Physical Medicine and Rehabilitation*,

Kiel, J. (1983) *Basic Hand Splinting. A Pattern Designing Approach*, Little Brown and Company.

Kielhofner, G. (1982) Theoretical Foundations of Occupational Therapy, *Proceedings of 8th International Congress of the World Federation of Occupational Therapists*, **2**, 1265–72.

Kielhofner, G. (1985) *A Model of Human Occupation, Theory and Application*, Williams and Wilkins, Baltimore, pp. 3–4.

Landau North, M. and Duddy, S. (1985) *Self-Help Through the Looking Glass*, Leicester Council for Voluntary Services.

Locker, D. (1983) *Disability and Disadvantage, the consequences of chronic illness*, Tavistock Publications, London, pp. 131–5.

Liang, M. and Jette, A. (1981) Measuring Functional Ability in Chronic Arthritis: a critical review, *Arthritis and Rheumatism*, **24**, 80–6.

Lorish, C., Parker, J. and Brown, S. (1985) Effective patient education, *Arthritis and Rheumatism*, **28** (11), 1289–97.

Mechanic, D. (1977) Illness Behaviour, Social Adaptation and the Management of Illness: A Comparison of Educational and Medical Models, *Journal of Nervous and Mental Diseases*, **165** (2), 79–87.

Meenan, R., Yelin, E., Nevitt, M. and Epstein, W. (1981) The impact of chronic disease, a sociomedical profile in rheumatoid arthritis, *Arthritis and Rheumatism*, **24** (3), 544–9.

Meenan, R. (1982) The Arthritis Impact Measurement Scales: Further Investigations of a Health Status Measure, *Arthritis and Rheumatism*, **25** (9), 1048–53.

Melvin, J. (1977) *Rheumatic Diseases: Occupational Therapy and Rehabilitation*, F.A. Davis Company.

Melzack, R. (1975) The McGill Pain Questionnaire: Major properties and scoring methods, *Pain*, **1**, 277–99.

Melzack, R. and Ward, P. (1982), *The Challenge of Pain* 2nd edn, Penguin Books, London, p. 60.

Melzack, R. and Wall, P. (1982) *The Challenge of Pain* Penguin Books, London, p. 222 and pp. 234–6.

Mosey, A. (1986) *Psychosocial Components of Occupational Therapy*, Raven Press, New York.

Naidoo, J. (1986) Limits to Individualism, in *The Politics of Health Education* (eds S. Rodmell and A. Watts) Routledge and Keagan Paul, London.

Nelson Jones, R. (1988) *Practical Counselling and Helping Skills* 2nd edn, Cassel, London, pp. 13–14.

Oakes, T., Ward, J., Gray, R., Klauber, M. and Moody, P. (1970) Family expectations and arthritis patient compliance to a hand resting splint regime, *Journal of Chronic Disability*, **22**, 757–64.

Pavlou, M., Harting, M. and Davis, F. (1978) Discussion groups for medical patients, *Psychotherapy and Psychosomatics* **30**, 105–15.

Pearlin, L. and Schooler, C. (1978) The structure of coping, *Journal of Health and Social Behaviour*, **19**, 2–21.

Potts, M., Weinberger, M. and Brandt, K. (1984) Views of patients and providers regarding the importance of various aspects of an arthritis treatment programme, *The Journal of Rheumatology*, **11** (1), 71–5.

Richardson, A. (1984) *Working With Self-Help Groups: A Guide for Professionals*, Bedford Square Press.

Rimon, L. (1985) Life stress and rheumatoid arthritis, *Psychotherapy and Psychosomatics*, **43** (1), 38–43.

Ritchie, D., Boyle, J. and McInnes, J. Clinical Studies with an Articular Index for the Assessment of Joint Tenderness in Patients with Rheumatoid Arthritis, *Quarterly Journal of Medicine*, **37**, 393–406.

Rogers, M., Laing, M. and Partridge, A. (1982) Psychological care of adults with rheumatoid arthritis, *Annals of Internal Medicine*, **96**, 344–8.

Shearer, A. (1981) *Disability: Whose Handicap?*, Blackwell, Oxford.

Seiger, M. (1984) Splints, Braces and Casts, in *Rheumatic Diseases, Rehabilitation and Management* (eds G. Riggs, E. Gall) Butterworth Publishers, London.

Shapriro-Slonaker, (1984) Joint Protection and Energy Conservation, in *Rheumatic Diseases, Rehabilitation and Management*, (eds G. Riggs, E. Gall) Butterworth Publishers, Guildford, p. 256.

Smiles, S. (1958) *Self-Help, with illustrations of Character, Conduct and Perseverance*, Centenary edition.

Smith-Pigg, J., Webb, P., Driscoll, W. and Caniff, R. (1985) *Rheumatology Nursing, A Problem Oriented Approach*, Wiley Medical Publications, Oxford, p. 115–7 and pp. 132–5.

Smith-Pigg, J., Webb, P., Driscoll, W. and Caniff, R. (1985) *Rheumatology nursing, a problem-oriented approach*, J. Wiley and Sons, Oxford, pp. 284–6.

Spiegel, J., Hirshfield, M. and Spiegel, T. (1985) Evaluating Self-Care Activities: Comparison of a Self-Reported Questionnaire with an Occupational Therapist interview, *British Journal of Rheumatology*, **24**, 357–61.

Steinbrocker, O., Traeger, C.and Battherman, R. (1949) Therapeutic criteria in rheumatoid arthritis, *Journal of American Medical Association* **140** 659–62.

Townsend, P. and Davidson, N. (1982) *Inequalities in Healthcare*, Penguin Books, London.

Trombly, C.A. (1983) *Occupational Therapy for Physical Dysfunction*, 2nd edn, Williams and Wilkins, Baltimore/London.

World Health Organization (WHO) (1980) *The international classification of impairments, disabilities and handicaps – a manual of classifications relating to the consequences of disease*, WHO Geneva.

Index

Relevant figures are indicated by page numbers in italics